The International Library of Psychology

THE WORLD OF COLOUR

Founded by C. K. Ogden

The International Library of Psychology

COGNITIVE PSYCHOLOGY
In 21 Volumes

THE WORLD OF COLOUR

DAVID KATZ

First published in 1935 by
Routledge, Trench, Trubner & Co., Ltd.

Reprinted in 1999 by
Routledge

2 Park Square, Milton Park, Abingdon, Oxfordshire OX14 4RN
711 Third Avenue, New York, NY 10017
First issued in paperback 2014

Routledge is an imprint of the Taylor and Francis Group, an informa business

Transferred to Digital Printing 2007

© 1935 David Katz
Translated from the German by R B MacLeod and C W Fox

British Library Cataloguing in Publication Data
A CIP catalogue record for this book
is available from the British Library

The World of Colour
ISBN 978-0-415-20961-8 (hbk)
ISBN 978-1-138-00739-0 (pbk)

Cognitive Psychology: 21 Volumes
ISBN 978-0-415-21126-0
The International Library of Psychology: 204 Volumes
ISBN 978-0-415-19132-6

CONTENTS

CONTENTS

PART III

SURFACE COLOURS

Chapter I. Achromatic Surface Colours in Achromatic Illumination

PART VI

COLOUR-CONSTANCY AND COLOUR-CONTRAST

PART VII

MEASURES OF THE PERCEPTION OF ILLUMINATION

PART VIII

COLOUR-CONSTANCY AND THE PROBLEM OF DEVELOPMENT

PART IX

THEORIES OF COLOUR-CONSTANCY

PREFACE TO THE ENGLISH EDITION

THE first edition of this book appeared in 1911, and the second in 1930. The occasion of the present translation was a suggestion made by Dr. R. H. Thouless of Glasgow. It was his opinion that the English reading public contains many who are interested in problems of colour, and that such a translation would serve to acquaint these more fully than has hitherto been possible with the type of problem treated in my book. I am grateful to Dr. Thouless not only for the suggestion but also for the keen interest with which he has followed the work of translation to its completion.

The publishers found it necessary to stipulate that the book be considerably abridged in translation. This caused me some misgivings at first, but I finally decided to undertake the task. During the preparation of the book for translation it became clear that many of the methods used in the original investigation have since then found general acceptance, and for this reason would no longer need to be presented in detail. On the same basis it proved feasible to omit many more or less intricate arguments for theses which are now considered as fairly well established and to reduce the number of references to the earlier literature.

I am particularly grateful to my good friend Dr. R. B. MacLeod for undertaking the tedious and time-consuming task of translation. Dr. MacLeod is one of those who understand the problems of colour-constancy best, and has himself made a significant experimental contribution.

I am also deeply indebted to Dr. C. W. Fox, who shared the work with him.

I should like, too, to express my warmest thanks to all those who during this period of great stress have made it possible for me to stay in Manchester, and in that way have assisted in the preparation of this translation.

FROM THE PREFACE TO THE SECOND
GERMAN EDITION

SINCE the appearance of the first edition of this book
nineteen years have passed. If. during this long period
it has not become as out of date as one might have
expected from a book of predominantly empirical character, I consider it as having been due not to me, but rather
to the fundamental method which I employed; and
no one could wish for a finer confirmation of the validity
of a method. This method is that of the unbiased
description of phenomena, to which the term " phenomenological method " is commonly applied.

Here and there the opinion has been expressed that
in the first edition the construction of theory did not
keep step with the presentation of factual material. I
am inclined to think, however, that such critics have
somewhat underestimated the amount of theory that
really is contained in the first edition. It must be granted,
I feel, that in a period when the whole of psychology
was still immersed in the gloom of atomistic dogma, to
have set up a totality theory of the perception of illumination and of the underlying physiological processes
is a theoretic achievement of some worth. It is not to
be regarded as a mere accident that Koffka himself, one
of the founders of the Gestalt theory, wrote in a review
of the first edition : " The significance of Katz's experiments . . . will reveal itself in the effects which the
work is bound to exercise on the whole field of psychological research." Even if the first edition was not
altogether untheoretical, I confess that I was in general
somewhat diffident about theorizing; and with good
grounds. The wealth of discovered fact was so great,

and its structure so many sided, that it was not easy to arrive at a single set of theoretical principles which would be valid for the whole. One cannot overlook the fact that all the attempts that have as yet been made to find a theoretical basis for the questions treated here suffer more or less from the drawback that they take only parts of the field into account, and fail to comprehend the whole. All the new facts and theories which seemed to me to be valuable have been incorporated, and have received ready recognition. Whoever desires in future to do work on the problem of colour-constancy will not need to go through the whole literature again, for I hope that nothing of significance has escaped my notice.

In view of the progress which has been made in the study of these problems, it seemed possible for me to make some more positive contributions to the theory. The direction I have taken corresponds in part with that indicated by the researches of other investigators. It corresponds, too, however, with the direction which my own thinking has been taking quite independently, and which expresses a developmental tendency evident in some of my more recently published works, particularly in my comprehensive work on the world of touch. The relationship between that work and this is evident even in the change of name which this book has undergone in the present edition.[1] Stated simply, my own development has been in the direction of according less and less significance to the influence of experience. Actually the first edition contains more evidence *against* the significance of individual experience than *for* it.

[1] The first edition appeared in 1911 as *Die Erscheinungsweisen der Farben und ihre Beeinflussung durch die individuelle Erfahrung*; the second in 1930 as *Der Aufbau der Farbwelt*.

GLOSSARY

The following German terms have been used in a more or less technical sense in the original. In some cases the English equivalents are by no means satisfactory, but were accepted simply because they have become current.

Ausgeprägtheit = pronouncedness.

Beleuchtung = illumination (as a phenomenal datum, or as a physical process).

Berücksichtigung der Beleuchtung = the taking into account of the illumination. ("Discounting the illumination" and "abstraction of the illumination" have been used by some writers.)

eigentliche Farbe = genuine colour.

Eindringlichkeit = insistence.

Erleuchtung = lighting (as a phenomenal datum, usually used with reference to the phenomenal lighting of space).

Erscheinungsweise = mode of appearance.

Farbmaterie, Farbwert = colour-matter (as distinguished from mode of appearance).

Flächenfarbe = film colour.

Glanz = lustre.

leuchtende Farbe = luminous colour.

Lochfarbe, Lochschirm = aperture-colour, aperture-screen.

Oberflächenfarbe = surface colour.

Raumfarbe = volume colour. (Many writers have used the term "bulky colour.")

subjektives Augengrau = subjective visual grey, intrinsic visual grey, subjective grey. (The term "cortical grey" used by some writers savours of theory rather than of description. Also, the term should not be confused with "ideo-retinal light" or "intrinsic light of the retina.")

Zwischenmedium = space-filling medium.

LIST OF ABBREVIATIONS FOR SOME OF THE WORKS CITED

K. Bühler, " Die Erscheinungsweisen der Farben," *Handbuch der Psychologie*, I. Teil. Die Struktur der Wahrnehmungen. Jena, 1922. =Bühler.

W. Fuchs, " Experimentelle Untersuchungen über das simultane Hintereinandersehen auf derselben Sehrichtung," *Zsch. f. Psychol.*, 1923, 91. =Fuchs I.

—— " Experimentelle Untersuchungen über die Aenderung von Farben unter dem Einfluss von Gestalten," *Zsch. f. Psychol.*, 1923, 92.

A. Gelb, " Die ' Farbenkonstanz ' der Sehdinge," *Handbuch der normalen und pathologischen Physiologie*, 12, 1929. =Gelb.

H. v. Helmholtz, *Vorträge und Reden*, Band 2, 4. Aufl. Braunschweig, 1896. =Helmholtz I.

—— *Handbuch der physiologischen Optik*, 2. Aufl. Hamburg and Leipzig, 1896. =Helmholtz II.

E. Hering, *Beiträge zur Physiologie.* Leipzig, 1861. =Hering I.

—— *Zur Lehre vom Lichtsinn.* Wien, 1878. =Hering II.

—— " Der Raumsinn und die Bewegungen des Auges," in Hermann's *Handbuch der Physiologie*, 3, Teil 1. Leipzig, 1879. =Hering III.

—— " Ueber die Theorie des simultanen Kontrastes von Helmholtz," *Pflügers Arch.*, 1888, 43. =Hering IV.

—— " Ueber das sogenannte Purkinjesche Phänomen," *Pflügers Arch.*, 1895, 60. =Hering V.

—— " Zur Lehre vom Lichtsinn," reprinted from Gräfe-Sämisch's *Handbuch der gesamten Augenheilkunde*, Teil 1, Kap. 12. Leipzig, 1905 and 1907. =Hering VI.

W. Metzger, " Optische Untersuchungen am Ganzfeld," *Psychol. Forsch.*, 1929, 13. =Metzger I.

G. E. Müller, " Zur Psychophysik der Gesichtsempfindungen," *Zsch. f. Psychol.*, 1896, 10. =Müller I.

—— " Zur Psychophysik der Gesichtsempfindungen," *Zsch. f. Psychol.*, 1897, 14. =Müller II.

—— *Ueber die Farbenempfindungen. Psychophysische Untersuchungen.* Leipzig, 1930. =Müller III.

The World of Colour

PART I

MODES OF APPEARANCE OF COLOUR AND THE PHENOMENOLOGY OF ILLUMINATION

§ 1. INTRODUCTION

IF we were to attempt to give a simple description of what the eye in its everyday activity tells us, we should have to do it somewhat as follows. We see objects of all sorts, some far away, some near at hand. An inexhaustible wealth of shapes and structures meets the eye, and when we attempt to give them some sort of systematic classification, we tend to do so on the basis of some such distinction as that of the natural and the artificial. Whether objects are located in the immediate vicinity or miles away from us, we always perceive between ourselves and the objects an empty space in which no objects are to be found. Everything that is visible has certain colour-properties, even if in individual cases it is not always easy for us to find the appropriate colour-names. With the same immediacy with which we perceive the colours of objects comes the apprehension of their illumination; and the illumination is not limited to the objects alone, for the empty space between objects is also seen as illuminated. It is important for our practical commerce with objects that we be able not only to perceive them but also to recognize the material of which they are composed, whether they be made of wood, paper, metal or other material. When objects are close at hand, we recognize their composition from the finer structures of the material which are then visible; at

A   I

greater distances, however, these means are no longer serviceable, and the eye has to make use of other criteria. The simple description of visual perception attempted here would not be complete without a reference to the fact that movement is normally present in the visual field. Objects can move from point to point in space, or movements can take place in objects.

The various aspects of visual perception to which reference has just been made represent distinct fields of psychological investigation, each with its correspondingly different methods. These branches concern themselves with the perception respectively of shape, of structure, of space, of colour and of movement. The studies reported in this book belong to the field of colour-perception, and it is our plan to pursue all the phenomena of visual perception which have anything to do with colour. Our interest in colour is not the interest of the physicist, nor again is it with those aspects of colour which puzzle the physiologist. Our concern is rather with the purely psychological problems of colour. From the psychological point of view, the field of colour includes also all our experiences of illumination, not the field of illuminating techniques but rather that of actually perceived illumination. The world as optic-æsthetic experience draws its beauty from the marvellous co-operation of colour-substance and illumination. Even if we are not going to be concerned with the spatial structure as such of the world, we shall have to consider spatial factors as they bear on colour. Inasmuch as space is always presented in coloured form, it plays an important part in determining the colour-impressions which we receive. Without the spatial factor we should lack the wealth of spatially organized modes of appearance which colours assume, and inasmuch as colour is always presented in spatial form it exercises a corresponding influence on the impression of space. Illumination operates as a creator and a destroyer of space ; even in the experience of empty space itself we see it as the really determining factor. Our study is not a study of configurations, but it must take into account the reciprocal relations which obtain between configurations, macrostructures and microstructures, and colour. Although it is not our intention to analyse the perception of movement, we shall have occasion to observe how significant an influence movement has on the phenomena of colour in connection with the interpenetration of colour and space.

Where do we encounter colours ? First of all they are certainly to be observed in objects. A paper is white, a leaf is green, coal is black. These are perfectly respectable experiences of colour which present us with no unusual problems. Then further : the sky is grey, the water has a green shimmer, and the air is full of beams of light. Such judgments, too, have to do with colour, and they seem to be perfectly commonplace. They involve the recognition of colours as objective properties, referred to objects in the environment. The attitude which dominates such judgments of colour we shall term the "natural," and, because of its significance for everyday life, the "biological" attitude. It is quite certain that people, with the exception of an insignificant fraction, have never dealt with colours except in this natural-biological way ; and animals depart from the biological attitude in their behaviour toward colour even less frequently than do men. Experiences of colour in their natural unbroken meaningfulness arise out of the need for a practical orientation toward the colour-qualities of the surrounding world. If the psychologist is rightly to envisage the problems set for him by the world of colour, he has to accept these tangible realities of the world of perception as his starting-point. It would be a kind of psychological perversion if he were to cast these cases aside, and, instead, begin his study with colour-phenomena which the colour specialist has been able to produce only under the highly artificial conditions of the laboratory. Most people depart from this world without ever having had a chance to look into an expensive spectroscope, and without ever having observed an after-image as anything other than as something momentarily

wrong with the eye.   Where is the man who of his own
accord would choose the subjective visual grey as an object
for observation ?   There was a time, nevertheless, when it
was primarily such phenomena as these which were accepted
as the only visual phenomena really worth studying.

Naturally the psychologist has no right to rest content
with the determination and description of colour-impressions, and assume that thereby all his work has been
completed.   That would be too easy.   His work must
begin with description, but it must also include the
attempt to detect relationships between phenomena and
underlying physical, physiological and psychophysical
processes.   The science of to-day is at least as much
interested in the genetic problem of " whence " as it is
in the problem of " what," and for that reason full justice
must be accorded to the point of view of developmental
psychology.

The naïve individual, dominated by the natural attitude,
deals with colours as properties of the objects of his
environment, not with colours as anything in the nature
of subjective experiences.   " In general the individual
gives no account of the colour which he has just seen.
He never makes colour an object of special consideration,
but uses it rather simply as a sign by the aid of which
objects are recognized."[1]   This is particularly evident,
as one might expect, among primitive people.   It was
Rivers who discovered the fact that as long as the colours
presented have primarily æsthetic value and no practical
significance, as in the case of the colours of the sky and
of vegetation, primitive people seem to be quite indifferent
to them.[2]   The Kaffir language alone has more than
twenty-six terms to designate the colour and markings
of horned cattle.[3]   According to Reche the Maori has approximately three thousand separately designated colours

[1] Hering, VI, p. 11.
[2] W. H. R. Rivers, Reports of the Cambridge Anthropological Expedition
to Torres Straits, 2, Physiology and Psychology.   Part I, Introduction and
Vision.   Cambridge, 1901, p. 96.
[3] H. Magnus, Untersuchungen über den Farbensinn der Naturvölker.
Jena, 1880, p. 19 ff.

which have practical significance for him.[1] In striking agreement with these facts of folk psychology is the observation of Gelb and Goldstein that, in cases of pathological absence of the indicative function of language, the experience of colour undergoes a reversal in the direction of a more concrete type of perception, closer to life and biologically more primitive.[2]

It is impossible to describe the totality of colour-phenomena without at the same time neglecting all other points of view from which colours might be studied. If one is to accomplish such a task one has to adhere rigorously and exclusively to the descriptive phenomenological point of view. No one ever realized how necessary such a procedure is for scientific precision more clearly than did Hering.[3] The modes of appearance of colour in space and the phenomena of illumination stand central in the studies reported in this book. The fact that illumination could in any sense at all be considered an independent psychological problem was not recognized until a phenomenologically trained eye was directed toward illumination as an independent *phenomenon*. So far as the modes of appearance of colour in space are concerned, the student of the psychology of colour has been in the habit of concentrating on the problem of colour alone, and consigning modes of appearance to the tender mercies of the student of space-psychology. And the student of space, on the other hand, has usually been too little interested in colours to accord them the attention they deserve. This hybrid position, in which the problem of " the modes of appearance of colours in space " seems to find itself, does not necessarily hold for the present study, since we shall concern ourselves first of all with this borderland between space and colour.

---

[1] E. Reche, *Tangaloa, ein Beitrag zur geistigen Kultur der Polynesier.* Munich and Berlin, 1926.

[2] *Psychol. Forsch.*, 1924, 6.

[3] " If anything is to be recognized as completely and definitely established as a result of Hering's efforts, it is the necessity for the psychological or, better stated, the phenomenological point of departure in colour theory." C. Stumpf, " Die Attribute der Gesichtsempfindungen," *Abhandlungen d. preuss. Akademie. d. Wiss. Phil.-hist. Kl.*, 1917, No. 8.

It would never occur to a writer on the psychology of colour to prove experimentally the validity of such relationships as the grouping of colours on the colour circle, for this system can be grasped only descriptively. In such a connection he is content simply to point to the experiences of colour which everyone of us has. In such cases experimental controls can serve only to render possible a clear presentation of the colour-experiences to which the writer is referring, and their discussion in connection with colour-experiences referred to in other studies. Neither here nor anywhere else can the psychologist produce new phenomena in the strict sense of the term ; what he does is simply to make mental phenomena speak for themselves, and in this way bring them to " official " recognition.

All experiments on colour which have not, like animal experiments, a pronouncedly behaviouristic character make some use or other of the medium of language. The interaction between colour-impression and linguistic expression is by no means of such a perfectly harmless character that the experimental results are thereby completely uninfluenced. The influences of language that are actually present are partly of a more or less external nature, partly, however, of a very fundamental kind, such as the relationships which obtain between language on the one hand, and sensation, ideation and thinking on the other. As far as the more external influences are concerned, all the difficulties arise which one encounters anywhere in the use of language. G. E. Müller's preface to his experiments on galvanic visual sensations is worth rereading in this connection.[1] Recently Jenny König has pointed out that we may speak of significant agreement in the naming of colours only with great reservations.[2] Such distortions of the perceptual process as those induced by language can be corrected. Another difficulty, however, is more deeply rooted, namely that which is grounded in the unavoidable lack

[1] G. E. Müller, *Zsch. f. Psychol.*, 1897, 14, p. 341 ff.
[2] Jenny König, *Arch. f. d. ges. Psychol.*, 1927, 60.

of correspondence between our linguistic resources and the ways in which the perceptual world is apprehended and articulated. It cannot be asserted that the consciousness of this situation is as lively in psychology as one would wish it to be, in view of its possible productivity as a psychological problem in itself. Valuable preliminary research has already been contributed by comparative linguistics. H. Güntert has repeatedly drawn attention to the fact that " language has played a very significant rôle in determining the constitution of man's spiritual world and in shaping his world of sense." [1] This borderland between sense-perception and linguistics has received particularly striking mention in numerous works of Weisgerber.[2] Henning in his book on smell gives considerable space to the linguistic factor. A particularly important contribution to the clarification of the relationships between colour-perception and linguistic expression is contained on the analysis by Gelb and Goldstein of the afore-mentioned case of amnesia for colour-names.

§ 2. How Colours appear in Space : The Modes of Appearance

Film Colours and Surface Colours.—It has always been clear to me that when one looks through the eyepiece of a spectroscope the colours one sees in it have an entirely different mode of appearance from that of other colours, *e.g.*, the colours of the coloured papers which we use so frequently.

The spectral colour of the usual apparatus is generally not localized so precisely at an exactly definable distance as is the colour of a paper. The latter usually appears wherever we see the surface of the paper. The distance of the spectral colour from the eye of the observer can be gauged only with some degree of uncertainty. The

[1] H. Güntert, *Wörter und Sachen*, Vol. IX, p. 6.
[2] L. Weisgerber (a) " Der Geruchsinn in unseren Sprachen," *Indogermanische Forschungen*, 1928, 46. (b) *Muttersprache und Geistesbildung*, Göttingen, 1929. (c) "*Adjektivische und verbale Auffassung der Gesichtsempfindungen*," *Wörter und Sachen*, 1929, 12.

absolute distance at which the spectral colour is presented is not to be held responsible for its peculiar mode of appearance. In the apparatus which I used (Asher's spectrometer) the distance at which the colours appeared varied according to the observer's estimate from 50 cm. to 80 cm. Now coloured papers can be presented at smaller or at greater distances without being thereby made to look like spectral colours. The variation which we observe in spectral colours with respect to ease of localization is connected in general with a certain spongy texture which they evince, whereas in the case of the colour of a paper we can speak of a greater compactness of the colour base. The paper has a surface in which the colour lies. The plane in which the spectral colour is extended in space before the observer does not in the same sense possess a surface. One feels that one can penetrate more or less deeply *into* the spectral colour, whereas when one looks at the colour of a paper the surface presents a barrier beyond which the eye cannot pass. It is as though the colour of the paper offered resistance to the eye. We have here a phenomenon of visual resistance which in its way contributes to the structure of the perceptual world as something existing in actuality.[1] The spongy texture of the spectral colour is not of such a nature that it could be referred to as a *voluminousness* or as a colour-*transparency*. Rather, a spectral colour has this much in common with the colour of a paper, that *it is extended through space in the form of a bi-dimensional plane, and functions as a rear boundary for it.* The delimitation of space takes place differently for the two types of colour. A spectral colour never loses an essentially *frontal-parallel* character. When the colour fixated is directly before the eyes, and projected on the fovea, the plane in which it is seen always presents an orientation essentially perpendicular to the direction of vision. The colour of a paper, on the other hand, can assume *any orientation whatsoever with reference to the*

---

[1] *Cf.* in this connection W. Dilthey, " Ueber die Gründe unseres Glaubens an die Existenz der Aussenwelt," *Berichte d. preuss. Akad. d. Wiss.*, 1890.

direction of vision, for its plane is always that of the surface of the coloured paper. If it appears in frontal-parallel orientation, this is to be considered simply as a special case. We shall distinguish between these two opposed types of colour-impression on the basis of their common and differentiating factors by characterizing spectral colours, and all the colours which share their mode of appearance, as *film colours* and the opposite type as *surface colours.* Surface colours are seen almost solely on objects, so that it might not be out of place to speak of them as " object colours."[1] In some cases, however, this term might be misleading. Thus we tend to consider the redness of a red glass or of a red liquid as an object colour, belonging to the object, whereas this red does not possess the character of a surface colour, but presents rather the mode of appearance which we shall characterize below as *voluminousness.*[2] On the other hand, surface colours do not appear only on objects ; they may be seen, for instance, on clouds of smoke or steam which stand out in clear relief, and we should be doing violence to common usage if we were to refer to these clouds of smoke or steam as objects.

Most naturally or artificially coloured objects, such as wood, paper, stone or cloth, awaken under ordinary conditions the impression of surface colour. By far the most common setting for this type of impression is when light is reflected diffusely from dull-surfaced objects, for as a rule it is only solidly structured objects which possess a clear-cut surface character. The relationship between the physical origin of a light-ray and the mode of appearance of the corresponding impression is not in accordance with any simple law. All possible inter-

[1] Wittmann has drawn attention to the fact that the colours of objects which are seen as reversed may present a decidedly surfacy character without actually being seen as object colours. J. Wittmann, *Arch. f. d. ges. Psychol.*, 1919, 39. Some further observations of surface, film and volume colours under similar conditions are reported by E. v. Hornbostel, *Psychol. Forsch.*, 1921, 1.

[2] " Thus we see that colour-impressions can constitute object colours of differing spatial mode of appearance." A. Gelb, " Ueber den Wegfall der Wahrnehmung von ' Oberflächenfarben,' " *Zsch. f. Psychol.*, 1920, 84, p. 245.

mediate stages are to be found between surface colours and film colours.[1] Monocular observation instead of the customary binocular observation results in a recession of surface colour. Lack of sharpness in accommodation can have the same effect. The surface colour-impression normally given by an object can easily be supplanted by the impression of film colour if a screen, containing a single aperture, is so placed before the object as to conceal it completely, except for the part appearing through the aperture, and at the same time to prevent the recognition of any surface structure in the object. Colour-impressions do not, however, change their modes of appearance only in response to changes in the external conditions. There are also more or less controllable inner sets which can bring about transformations of colour-appearance. Some observations made by v. Allesch [2] are worth quoting in this connection. " It often happened that the same colour appeared at one time as surface colour, at another as film and at yet another as volume colour. . . . The purposeful set of the observer [was] in this connection of great significance." It is noteworthy that the transformation from surface colour to film colour is more easily induced than is the reverse change. Even the transformation of film colour into volume colour " was not altogether as obvious and as easy as the opposite." We chose spectral colours as our original example of film colours; nevertheless any physical light-ray can produce the impression of film colour. A blue or uniformly beclouded grey sky presents an opportunity for the observation of film colours. If one wishes to limit

[1] G. E. Müller has drawn attention to the fact that a visual phenomenon tends of its own accord to approximate more closely the mode of appearance of film and volume colours the more closely its intensity approximates that of the intrinsic visual grey. *Zsch. f. Sinnesphysiol.*, 1923, 54, p. 140. " Reds and yellows certainly possess the property of being more strongly condensed, whereas the colours on the right half of the spectrum are blurred." Sophie Belajew-Exemplarsky, *Zsch. f. Psychol.*, 1925, 96, p. 424. Mabel F. Martin has made a special study of transitional stages between film, surface and volume colours " Film, Surface and Bulky Colours and their Intermediates," *Amer. J. Psychol.*, 1922, 33.
[2] G. J. v. Allesch, *Die ästhetische Erscheinungsweise der Farben*. Berlin, 1925, p. 22.

oneself to a relatively small section of the sky one can use an aperture screen. If one lies on one's back in a large open meadow, and looks upward, the sky produces the impression of a very extended film colour. In connection with the localization of film colours with reference to the aperture in the screen through which it is seen, exhaustive experiments will be reported below (§ 12). For me the intrinsic visual grey also approximates the film-colour appearance. According to my experiments this proves to be the case for other individuals as well, but a number of people have classified it rather as a volume colour. The intensity of illumination within a given space can be so reduced that it becomes impossible, even with a completely adapted eye, to recognize either the structure or the orientation of the surfaces of objects. What can still be distinguished are merely the outlines of objects and those of their surfaces which stand out as distinct from each other on the basis of brightness differences. The grey colours perceived under these conditions resemble film colours.

The "indefinite localization" of a film colour implies for us a positive statement about its localization. The expression is used in a purely descriptive sense. We shall encounter later, too, the experiences of "indefinite" illumination and "indefinite" colour. The category of indefiniteness seems to deserve greater consideration in the psychology of perception (and in other fields as well) than it has as yet been accorded. Rubin deserves credit for having drawn attention to impressions of indefinite size and of indefinite configuration.[1]

We have seen that film colour always possesses an essentially frontal-parallel character. In contrast with this, surface colours *may* have an afrontal orientation, since they always lie in the surface of the object in which they are seen. Resulting from this peculiarity is a new factor which distinguishes surface colour further from film colour. The surface of an object can be either

[1] E. Rubin, *Visuell wahrgenommene Figuren*. Gyldendalske Boghandel, 1921, § 8.

smooth or wrinkled, and according as it is the one or the other the surface colour, too, will be either smooth or wrinkled. Surface colour follows all the wrinkles of the surface of the object, and presents, too, its finest structure and texture. Film colour, on the other hand, is always localized in a smooth plane. Pronounced wrinkles never appear in film colours. One might assume from this that greater pronouncedness of structure or texture would in itself be enough to stamp certain colour-impressions as surface colours ; where structure or texture is absent we should then have film colours. The distinction between surface and film cannot, however, be made as easily as this. If we stretch a sheet of exceedingly smooth paper, which is not shiny, across a pane of glass, and view it from a sufficiently great distance, we shall have a surface colour from which all texture is completely absent.

Not all colours which we see as colour-qualities of objects possess the character of surface colour, but it seems to hold fairly generally that all surface colours are seen as attributes of objects. Contrariwise it is not our custom in the same sense to associate with film colour the impression that it refers beyond to some sort of object. It appears simply as a " smooth or space-filling *quale*," as Hering[1] expressed it on one occasion when he had this particular mode of appearance in mind.

Some brief reference must be made to the different *æsthetic* effects of these two modes of appearance of colour. For most of the observers whom I have questioned in this connection the film colours have a certain delicacy about them, and for this reason are characterized as æsthetically more pleasing than the surface colours.[2]

This is the proper place for a discussion of a few

---

[1] Hering, VI, p. 12. Matthaei occasionally refers to film colour as " free colour." R. Matthaei, *Die Welt der Farbe*. Bonn, 1927. Free colour becomes condensed into surface colour or diffuses itself into volume colour.

[2] " Numerous special experiments . . . indicated that the specifically æsthetic appearance of colour is the film colour, a factor which comes into operation, too, when a coloured object is judged as far as possible on the basis of its colour alone (as is nowadays being attempted in impressionistic painting)." v. Allesch, *op. cit.*, p. 22.

observations reported by Gelb in that valuable article mentioned above on the disappearance of the perception of surface colours, in which my distinction between the different modes of appearance of colour received its first application to questions in the pathology of perception.

The study is of two cases of disturbance of colour-vision, brought about by cerebral lesion.[1] In each case the lesion was occipital. In the case of one of the patients, who because of his greater intelligence and reliability proved to be a particularly fruitful subject, the diagnosis was of a wound-scar " which indicated an original wound on the left side in the region of the inferior parietal lobe and of the lateral part of the occipital lobe." At the time of the investigation there was a total colour-blindness involving the whole visual field (but no central scotoma). Within approximately four months colour-sensitivity was almost completely restored. The brightness distribution in the spectrum corresponded exactly to that of the normal eye. At a certain stage in the course of recovery the patient proved on examination to be trichromatic for very large areas, dichromatic for areas of medium size and monochromatic for very small areas. In the achromatic stage the patient was not capable of voluntarily recalling memory images of previously seen colours, but apart from this colour-amnesia there was also at the beginning of the recovery period an amnesia for colour-names. We have thus a case of the loss of what we shall later discuss in detail under the heading of " memory colour " (§ 32). " We observed this lack of ability to recall colours, previously perceived in the normal state, in all of the patients with colour-disturbances resulting from a lesion at the cortical end of the optic tract " (p. 198). Gelb speaks here of an apperceptive mental blindness.

Now that we have presented the general facts of the case, we may proceed to a more detailed discussion of its

[1] Gelb refers to a similar case described by O. Pötzl, Die optisch-gnostischen Störungen, *Handbuch der Psychiatrie*, ed. by Aschaffenburg, Spez. Teil, 3 Abt., 2 Hälfte, 2 Teil, 1 Band. Leipzig and Vienna, 1928, pp. 158 and 238.

significance for the present investigation. " A more careful analysis of the perceptual process revealed the fact that the colours of visual objects assumed for the patient the character of film colours, having almost the appearance of volume colours." It was discovered that " the colours of all visual objects had for the patient lost their surfacy character, in the sense that as far as localization and spatiality were concerned they had in part assumed the character of film colours which came very close to being volume colours." The patient was unable to localize the colours of objects as definitely at a precisely reportable distance as a normal person could. Colours failed to lie flat on the surfaces of objects. The distance between the actual position of the surface of a paper and the position at which the patient localized it varied with the type of colour, being in general greater with bright than with dark colours. Colours appeared to the patient to have a spongy texture ; everything appeared " fuzzy and soft." The patient had to reach *into* the colour in order to touch the surface of a coloured object. He had to plunge farthest in when the paper was black and least when the paper was white. A coloured plate was " always apprehended in the frontal-parallel plane, whether its orientation was perpendicular or oblique to the direction of vision." According to Gelb " there can be no doubt that our patient had lost the ability to perceive surfaces." " All the spatial criteria which Katz sets up as being especially characteristic of film colours apply directly to the way in which the colours of objects in space appeared to our patient." In perfect agreement with what is said below (p. 67), Gelb observes that even his patient's filmy colour-impressions possess a relatively definite localization with reference to each other. As surface colour-perception was restored, it was the bright colours which first recovered their surface character.

Because of their significance with reference to the theoretical discussion which is to follow, I should like to report here some further observations of Gelb's in connection with the same case.   If the patient was presented with a series of greys, ranging from very dark to very light in steps approximating a normal scale of just noticeable differences, and was asked to indicate the number of brightness differences which he recognized in the whole series, he would point out only four steps. " He reported spontaneously that these four brightness steps represented *sharp breaks in continuity* " (p. 203). Thus the patient saw not a kind of regular, steeply mounting series, corresponding to the increase in brightness, but rather four distinct steps.   Gelb points out that the different " thicknesses " of the colours are not intelligible solely on the basis of their different degrees of insistence, since a white in weak illumination appeared thinner than a black which through a reduction screen[1] would appear the same as the white.   As long as the ability to see surface colours continued to be absent, the patient in characterizing his impressions always used the expressions " bright " and " dark," never the expressions " black " and " white."

There is also evidence to indicate the existence of numerous relationships between the differences which I have demonstrated among the various modes of appearance of colour and Rubin's well-known analyses of the figure-ground relationship.   Rubin found that " the colour of the ground approaches more closely the appearance of film colour than does the colour of that part of the field which is apprehended as figure " (p. 57).

Certain objections might be raised against what has been said.   It is true, one might say, that film and surface colours are different, but this difference does not have its basis in the colour-impression as such, but is connected rather with the multifarious influences of experience.   In so far as this objection is causal-genetic in character it does not concern us, since we have sought here simply to give an unbiassed description of phenomena as they appear.   The problem of the causal-genetic relationship between film and surface colours—in itself an important

[1] *Cf.* p. 55.

problem—must await later examination. An objection with reference to underlying principle might, however, be raised. Granted the difference between one mode of appearance and another, are not these differences irrelevant as far as the essence of colour-phenomena is concerned ? The acceptance of such a suggestion would commit one to the arbitrary selection of certain aspects of the factual material to be studied, and this selection would first have to be justified. For, since no colour is ever presented in experience without some kind of spatial characteristics, one would in such a case have either to limit one's study to colours of a single mode of appearance, and exclude colours of all other types, or simply to assert that the mode of appearance of a colour on any particular occasion is of no significance for the colour-impression. Such a delimitation, on the one hand, could not be adequately grounded, and we shall have occasion to demonstrate also that the alternative assertion does not fit the facts.

Fiedler has objected to my conception of the modes of appearance of colour on the ground that colours "possess in fact no mode of appearance at all," the characteristic being attributable only to objects.[1] In this connection F. Krueger writes : " But what Katz, accepting too hastily the support of Husserl's philosophy, has called modes of appearance of colours ought more properly speaking to be termed modes of appearance of things." According to this, Krueger would appear to be endorsing Fiedler's point of view. Having rejected the method which I have here adopted, Fiedler in his search for the only true colour-sensations concludes as follows : " Thus our experiments demonstrate unambiguously that black, grey and white cannot be sensations, cannot be elementary light qualities. . . . Psychologically simple experiences are the colourless quality, which is more or less bright or dark, and the colours of the . . . spectrum." It is a purely arbitrary assumption that it is

---

[1] K. Fiedler, *Neue psychol. Stud.*, 1926, 2, p.391. I have given a detailed criticism of Fiedler's article in my second critical review of studies in the field of visual perception. *Psychol. Forsch.*, 1929, 12.

precisely these colours, the colours which Fiedler accepts as his starting-point, which are " the " colour-sensations, that they represent that which is most primitive among colour-impressions. This attitude is altogether dogmatic. We must constantly emphasize the fact that visual sensations in Fiedler's sense are not psychical " reals " but are rather hypothetical constructs. In opposition to Fiedler one would emphasize anew the methodological necessity for a position which takes natural colour-experiences as its starting-point. This leads us directly into a study of the modes of appearance of colour.

Gelb remarks in one place that perhaps the doctrine of the attributes of sensation will have to undergo a reconstruction to take into account the modes of appearance of colour. With this I am in agreement. Stumpf, in his penetrating analysis of the problem, cited above, does not seem to me to be justified in his explicit exclusion of surface colours from consideration. The locus within the total realm of colours of colour-" sensations " (his point of departure) is not easy to determine.

Transparent Film, Surface and Volume Colours.—Let us hold a piece of smoked glass of medium transparency or a piece of coloured gelatine before us at arm's length in such a way that its boundaries are visible.[1] If, now, we look through it with both eyes at an object beyond, *e.g.*, at an open book, we believe that we can see the latter *through* the glass or the gelatine. The more naturally and freely we allow our fixation to wander, the clearer the impression is, whereas a pronouncedly critical attitude impairs it. The grey of the glass or the colour of the gelatine is localized in a plane which in many cases coincides approximately with the plane of the glass or gelatine itself. We shall refer to colours of this mode of appearance, which are seen in transparent objects, as *transparent film colours.* Any number and any gradation of transparent colours can be had when one looks through what is called an episcotister, a rotating chromatic or achromatic disc with an open sector of variable size.

[1] " If transparency is to be achieved the nearer (transparent) colour must also be configured, if only as a plane or film." Fuchs, I, p. 175.

Even a superficial study of transparent film colours enables one to recognize the following characteristics. As the name itself suggests, transparent film colours do not obscure the background. Through them objects can be seen, and as far as quality is concerned the surface colours of these objects are partially influenced by the transparent colour lying before them. It is highly doubtful if behind a *transparent* film colour one could ever have a *space-delimiting* film colour. If the latter is brought behind a transparent film colour both colour-impressions usually fuse in such a way that it becomes altogether impossible to separate them in perception. They appear rather as a film colour bounding approximately that section of space in which the film colour or the transparent colour in itself was seen. If we view a blue or uniformly clouded sky monocularly through a coloured glass, we have the impression of a film colour of a tint corresponding to a combination of the colour of the sky and the colour of the glass. When we accommodate for the central part of the glass we localize the colour approximately at that distance, and when we accommodate for the sky itself it appears at a distance not quite as far away as that at which the sky is normally seen. The same fusion effect between transparent colour and what is normally seen as surface colour can be observed when an aperture is placed in such a way as to prevent the perception of the object which bears the surface colour. This is naturally bound up with the fact that the said surface colour has now taken on the character of a film colour. The transparency of a colour is clearer and most pronounced when the surface behind it is fixated binocularly. Under these conditions the surface colour evinces a tendency to assimilate the orientation of the transparent colour to its own. Transparent colours can also be observed in experiments on binocular colour-mixture, where the colour presented to one eye is seen to glimmer through the colour presented to the other eye. A great variety of transparent colours can be produced in the following manner. Fixate a particular point on a printed page with both eyes. Now introduce an opaque object of any colour whatsoever, *e.g.*, a cardboard, before one eye. This should be approximately half-way between the paper and the eye, and held in such a way that the binocularly fixated point is concealed from the eye. The impression thus created is as if the fixated point were seen through the colour of the opaque object. All phenomena of transparency achieved by these means (gelatine, smoked glass, episcotister, interposed cardboard) gain extraordinarily in clarity if the intermediate object is displaced with reference to the fixated point. "Under all experimental conditions movement of the head or of one object or even of both objects enhances the transparency greatly."[1] In another connection I have already pointed out that a striking increase in transparency is brought about when tissue-paper lying on a printed surface is set in motion, although it must be remembered that here certain physical as well as psychological conditions are favouring the production of transparency.[2]

Transparent colours obtained through the medium of objects which are in themselves opaque, *e.g.*, a cardboard, as in the experiment just described, may be distinguished from those obtained with the aid of a glass, a gelatine disc or an episcotister in that they present a texture derived from the texture of the opaque objects themselves, whereas because there is no texture in glass, gelatine or episcotister the transparent colours produced by these means do not present any texture either. If we characterize the latter as transparent film colours, we may refer to the colours produced with the assistance of the cardboard as *transparent surface colours*. In the

---

[1] Fuchs, I, p. 220.
[2] D. Katz, *Der Aufbau der Tastwelt*, Leipzig, 1925, p. 32. If with the assistance of two projection lanterns two colour patterns are exposed on a surface, and moved back and forth in opposite directions, " there can be seen several different patterns through each other when the colours are the same, and one pattern moving behind another when the colours are different, just as if we had two curtains one suspended behind the other." R. H. Goldschmidt, *Postulat der Farbwandelspiele*, Heidelberg, 1928, p. 40.

foregoing discussion the surface colours considered first were opaque. Opaque surface colours are so completely dominant in visual perception that it did not seem necessary to make explicit reference to their opaqueness even in designating them. In the discussion to follow, too, where reference is made to surface colours as such, the opaque variety will always be meant. At this point, however, a few more words should be said about transparent surface colours. Henning carried out a number of experiments on transparent surface colours, partly of the nature of the afore-mentioned experiment with the cardboard, and partly employing a stereoscopic technique. Instead of the cardboard he used objects with shiny surfaces or objects which were covered with print or could be illuminated in various ways. Some of Henning's conclusions are as follows : 1. Transparent colours can show lustre and surface structure. 2. When the illumination is changed, the transparent colour's own surface character does not undergo a qualitative change, but appears, rather, simply as differently illuminated. 3. Transparent colours are localized at a precisely determinable distance. 4. Surface colours are not bound down to a frontal-parallel mode of appearance. 5. It is possible behind the transparent colour to see a space-delimiting film colour.[1]

In everyday life we often have transparent surface colours when we look through panes of glass. "A plane surface whose outer limits we cannot see, and on which we can distinguish no spots, roughnesses, lines or superimposed objects, is not recognized as a surface; it remains as invisible as the surface of a mirror."[2] Most panes of glass with which we have to do in practical life do not, however, correspond to the transparent surface just described, but are noticeable because of the more or less systematic distortions of the objects seen through them. Their visibility becomes clearer when they are

[1] H. Henning, *Zsch. f. Psychol.*, 1921, 86.
[2] H. Cornelius, *Elementargesetze der bildenden Kunst.* Leipzig, 1908, p. 60.

overlaid with a deposit of tiny dust particles. The resulting cloudy effects, produced on the surface of the glass, combine to give the impression of a transparent plane, which we shall characterize as a *coherence-plane*, a term which Bühler[1] has used in a similar context. It is these cloudy effects which, taken together, really make the surface of the glass visible as a transparent surface colour. The impression of this transparent surface colour varies, too, with the intensity of the attendant illumination.

Related in some sense to transparent surface colours are *volume colours*, or colours which are seen as organized in and filling a tri-dimensional space. According to my observations they possess this property clearly only when they are at the same time genuinely *transparent*. A slightly cloudy liquid in a glass vessel seems to me to be genuinely voluminous only where I can discern objects through it. The space which appears as actually filled with colour is distinguished clearly from its surroundings in so far as objects can be seen behind it. Such colours with a voluminous mode of appearance are described by Hering.[2] The voluminousness of a fog is given clearly only as long as objects can be perceived through it. If the fog becomes so thick as seriously to impair the perception of objects, or if one directs his gaze in such a way that objects can no longer be seen through it, *e.g.*, if one looks at the sky, the voluminousness of the whitish colour disappears. The white which is still perceptible becomes then a limiting film colour. Under otherwise similar conditions the more one can see objects through a fog the more the thickness of the fog seems to recede. The question as to the extent to which clear air or, to express it differently, empty space is phenomenologically given will be considered in another context.

Mirrored Colours and Lustre.—When the surface of an object is smooth it reflects light according to a simple law. If the reflection is of such a nature that recognizable

[1] K. Bühler, *Die Erscheinungsweisen der Farben.* Leipzig, 1922, p. 60 ff. Hereafter cited as Bühler.
[2] Hering, III, p. 573 f. ; also Hering, VI, p. 11 f.

images of objects are produced in the eye, we speak of
the surface as having the properties of a *mirror*. If,
however, the images are not recognizable, and if instead
certain parts of the surface lose their surface structure
and appear as essentially brighter, we speak then of a
lustre which lies on the surface of the object. We may
distinguish between two types of mirroring. It may
take place in such a way that the proper colour of the
mirroring surface plays a diminishing rôle in determining
the colour of the image seen in the mirror. This is the
case, for instance, with mercury or silver mirrors. As
far as the mode of appearance of colours reflected in
mirrors of this kind is concerned, no problems of significance emerge. In such cases surface colour simply
remains surface colour, film colour remains film colour,
etc. The question as to how we distinguish between an
object and its reflection need not concern us here.[1]
When reflection is perfect, the reflecting surface itself
is not perceived. Thus we see mirrored objects in a
sense *behind* the reflecting surface but not, strictly
speaking, *through* it. We see through the surface when
the mirroring is of the second sort. If, for instance, the
colour of a mirroring surface is itself visible, the reflected
object is seen behind that surface but through the proper
colour of the surface. The colour of this surface is not
essentially different from the previously described transparent film colour ; it is merely easier for us to distinguish
the colour of the reflecting surface from that of the
reflected object, because of the greater uniformity of the
former, than to distinguish between transparent film
colour and the colour seen through it. The mirrored
colour-impression retains its independence to a greater
extent, *i.e.*, it is less influenced by the colour of the
mirror than a colour seen through a transparent medium
is influenced by the transparent film colour. The
difference in localization, too, between mirroring surface

---

[1] A pretty case bearing on the development of the mirror illusion in
people who have recovered sight after having been blind from birth is
reported by W. Uhthoff, *Zsch. f. Psychol.*, 1897, 14, p. 203 ff.

and mirrored colour is greater than the corresponding difference in the field of transparent film colours. The black mirror of the landscape painter is adapted to mirroring of the former kind. This consists of a plate of glass, which is covered with a black colour instead of with a sheet of metal. Chromatically coloured mirrors can be produced in the same way, if glass plates are interlaid with coloured paper, or if one side of a glass is painted with a saturated varnish. Polished wood, too, such as mahogany, affords an opportunity for observations of mirror effects such as those made by Helmholtz.[1]

Let us turn to the description of the phenomena of lustre.[2] The description of these phenomena is often confused with considerations of the conditions of their production. We shall find ourselves in essential agreement with Hering's position as expressed in his brief but pertinent remarks on the subject of lustre.[3] It is customary to distinguish between different kinds of lustre, e.g., metallic lustre, the lustre of silk, the lustre of graphite. Metallic lustre is, however, not confined merely to metals, nor is silky lustre confined merely to silks. These materials merely possess in particularly pronounced fashion the types of lustre to which their names have been given. It can be stated as a general law that lustre appears only on an object, and, as it exceeds in brightness the colour of the object and partially destroys its surface structure, it is apprehended as a light which does not really belong to the colour of the object.[4] Where lustre is seen objects are given, or at least appear to be given, as carrying the lustre. Clouds which are seen

---

[1] Helmholtz, II, p. 557 f., 563.
[2] A. Kirschmann, " Der Metallglanz und die Farbe der Metalle," *Arch. f. d. Ges. Psychol.*, 1921, 61.
[3] Hering, III, p. 576.
[4] " Lustre comes into being only when the light, which normally belongs to the mirrored object, is broken away from it, and appears to lie wholly or partially on the mirroring surface." " The phenomenon of the coherence-plane is necessary for the appearance of smoothness, the coherence-plane acting as the bearer of the surplus lustre-light." Bühler, pp, 159, 172. This is supported by the fact that a mirror can be made lustrous if lycopodium powder is scattered over it. C. Baumann, *Pflügers Archiv.*, 1902, 91.

as lustrous possess the illusory appearance of formed objects; the light that lies upon them is not seen as part of their proper colour. The lustre that plays on the surface of moving water is certainly not considered as the colour belonging to the water. In the great majority of cases the phenomena of lustre occur in connection with surface colours. The lustrous point itself, because of the afore-mentioned destruction of surface structure, never appears as a clear-cut surface colour, but in many respects resembles rather a film colour. Where light seems to be superimposed on a surface colour, the surface structure underneath the light remains perceptible. When intensity is greatly increased a film colour may become *luminous*, but it never becomes lustrous. Lustre-light does not lie *in* the plane of the object to which it belongs, but appears rather either *before* the object or *superimposed on* it. Mirror-images, on the other hand, are always localized *behind* the reflecting surface. This difference in localization of the surplus light of objects is in part responsible for the phenomenal difference between mirrored colour and lustre. The lustrous points of the objects always possess a surplus of brightness, which is seen as separate and distinct from the object colour. The lustrous points, however, need only be relatively bright, not bright in any absolute sense. " If something is sensed as brighter than objects which in the same illumination appear as pure white (and if the greater brightness cannot under the circumstances be apprehended as superimposed light) we see it as luminous or as lustrous."[1] This does not, however, hold for all cases. If we look at the lustre of a black silk hat we can easily convince ourselves that a piece of white paper placed in the same illumination beside the lustrous part of the hat appears much brighter. Or we may take as an example the lustre-lights on the human skin. They certainly do not possess the brightness of white paper under the same illumination. Undoubtedly the painter succeeds in many cases in representing lustre in his

---

[1] Hering, III, p. 575.

pictures without having to use the brightest colour on his palette, namely, white. This, however, cannot be considered as an argument against Hering, for pictorially represented space involves laws of illumination which are different from those which govern the space in which the picture is seen. The impression of lustre is not dependent on the presence at the lustrous point of light of any specific high intensity, a fact which becomes obvious when we realize that we can with the assistance of an episcotister reduce the amount of light reflected by a lustrous body to a few hundredths of its strength without diminishing its lustrous character. It is to be expected that binocular observation of lustrous objects will enhance the specific impression of lustre, because the difference in binocular parallax between the light diffusely reflected and the light directly reflected from the object makes the distinction between object colour and super-imposed light clearer. It is to be recognized, however, that lustre is also visible in monocular observation, pro-vided only that the requisite colour-experiences are produced. From this point of view it becomes intelligible that in monocular vision a movement of the head or of the object should enhance the impression of illumination.[1] On the one hand, these conditions favour the breaking up of the light into diffusely and directly reflected light, and, on the other hand, the movement permits the fulfilment of our expectation that the lustrous point will appear *also* in its proper colour, *i.e.*, in the object colour of the rest of the body. The lustre of objects and materials which are easily moved about is frequently referred to as glitter. If two marginless surfaces are presented stereoscopically, a white to one eye and a black to the other, the result is rivalry of visual fields or binocular colour-mixture. If, however, these colours are presented on surfaces which represent something with object character, *e.g.*, a glass object, a vivid impression of lustre

[1] Bühler calls attention to the fact that movement is not to be con-sidered as one of the indispensable conditions for the production of lustre, since according to Helmholtz's experiments lustre can be seen even when the object is momentarily illuminated. Bühler, p. 161.

may be aroused. A lustrous point can be immediately deprived of its lustrous character by any adjustment which conceals the object bearing the lustre. The afore-mentioned methods of reducing a surface colour to film colour are also effective in reducing lustre. Here, too, an aperture screen proves to be most effective. If the lustrous region of an object is viewed through such a screen the aperture is seen as filled with a film colour in which no trace of lustre is perceptible. If the object were exceedingly lustrous one might see the aperture as luminous, but the impartial observer would never be able to perceive any lustre. According to my observations lustre possesses in general an unstable character ; the more critically one regards it the more it recedes. When I observe monocularly, and with a special inner set, I can nearly always succeed, even without using a screen, in making the lustre appear as a luminous colour.

How are the different kinds of lustre to be distinguished from each other ? When we have a clear metallic lustre we can nearly always discern a *marked* brightness difference between the lustrous and the dull parts of the object. This great brightness difference is undoubtedly necessary for the production of a clear impression of metallic lustre. It is not in itself sufficient, however, for such differences in brightness may also be observed when the lustre is of a different kind. More significant seems to be the special configuration of the lustre-light. It displays greater uniformity in the case of metals than it does in connection with other kinds of lustre, *e.g.*, in the lustre of silk. The lustre-light in metallic lustre sometimes possesses the character of a thickness filling out space. Further is to be mentioned the fact that the lustre-light of a metal is presented against a colour ground of a very special mode of appearance. We can recognize *metallic surfaces as such* on the basis of their inner structure, even when we see only their non-lustrous or dully lustrous parts. It is impossible to select a grey which under a specified illumination is identical with the colour of the non-lustrous parts of a silver plate. Even in their non-lustrous or dully lustrous parts, metals do not appear as simple surface colours. We perceive the surface of the metal, it is true, but its colour seems to lie *behind* this surface. As in the case of film colour, we feel that we are boring through the surface into the colour of the metal. This mode of appearance is possessed by all metals or materials which have a metallic appearance. What is unique about metallic lustre lies accordingly less in the isolated colour-impression of the lustrous parts than in the colour-" configuration " which the lustrous and non-lustrous parts together constitute. Similarly what is unique about the other types of lustre is to be sought more in the way in which the lustre-lights appear against a background of colours than in any one peculiar structure.

Luminosity and Glow.—Hering was probably thinking of flames when, in addition to greater brightness, which we, too, hold to be essential, he considered voluminousness to be characteristic of luminosity.[1] For it happens not infrequently that we see luminous colours with a filmy organization. If in a room which is otherwise not illuminated, we focus a beam of light on one side of a translucent paper or milk-glass disc, the observer, looking at the other side, has the clear-cut impression of a *luminous film*, which is oriented fairly definitely with reference to him. If the light source is adjusted in such a way that it can be seen behind the paper or disc, or if in some other way the observer is made aware of its presence, he then tends to have the impression that the light is *shining through* or that the paper or disc is *self-luminous*. If coloured translucent paper is used in this experiment, the luminosity acquires a voluminous character. Colours which appear filmy or voluminous must exceed their surroundings in brightness if they are to produce the impression of luminous colour. The luminous appearance is dependent on the presence of a definite absolute light-intensity, so that even in an otherwise perfectly dark visual field a surface cannot appear as luminous until the light has exceeded a certain minimal

[1] Hering, III, p. 575.

strength. If the light emitted by a phosphorescent surface in a dark room is so weak that other objects are not thereby rendered visible, the impression created is that of a bright film colour in an otherwise dark visual field, but not that of a genuinely luminous film colour. The most useful criterion is that suggested by Hering, namely that a colour must be brighter than a white under the same conditions of illumination if it is to be characterized as luminous.[1] A flame which is presented in the visual field continues to appear luminous even when its intensity and that of the whole visual field are reduced by means of an episcotister to a few hundredths of the original intensity. The artist creates the illusion of a luminous object in a picture not so much by painting the object in particularly bright colours as by distributing the light and shadow appropriately with reference to the object within the pictorially represented space.

With Hering's description of the visual impressions of *glow* I am in complete agreement.[2] I might add that the impression of glow is to be distinguished from that of simple luminosity in that a glowing object is perceived as a more or less clearly defined figure, whereas no definite limits can be set for luminous flames. No sharp dividing line can, however, be drawn between the two impressions.

§ 3. TIME AND THE PHENOMENA OF COLOUR

In my book on touch I referred to the variations in the manner in which the temporal factor is presented to consciousness in impressions of different senses. " In a perfectly uniform tone, which is undergoing no qualitative or intensive change, we experience an uninterrupted rise and fall . . . we experience in the strict sense of the term a process . . . This temporal structure is not possessed by a colour-experience ; a colour which is

---

[1] Hering, III, p. 575.

[2] " A glowing piece of iron is seen as luminous throughout its mass." The red of iron which glows and radiates light " is seen not simply as film colour on its surface but as extending back into the object." Hering, III, p. 575.

presented in a stationary visual field neither comes into being nor disappears as does a tone ; . . . a colour is experienced as something permanently there." [1]   These remarks are not intended to imply that colour-phenomena are not affected in any way by processes operative in time. No reference need be made here to those changes in colours, occurring in time, which result from changes in illumination, or which are induced by changes in position with reference to light-source. It is probably customary to consider such colour-impressions as differing in no way from those presented in a stationary field apart from the fact that they are in temporal succession. If such were the case, a breaking-up of the impressions which was purely temporal in character would induce no change of any sort in them. We shall for the moment beg the question as to whether there are colour-experiences which, in keeping with this point of view, would actually remain quite unchanged, even if they were broken up into smaller temporal units. Our concern here is to demonstrate the fact that, at any rate, there are also some colour-experiences which require time and movement for their very existence, and which have no existence at all in a stationary field.

It was not difficult for me to demonstrate that in connection with the sense of touch there are phenomena which come into being exclusively in and through movement, in fact that almost all specific touch impressions are really born of movement. Our failure to recognize the multitude of such impressions, which we have, can be explained only as a result of the fact that we have fallen victim to a rigid experimental method, an experimental method which is itself rooted in a time atomism which represents one of the many forms of psychological atomism. Although this time atomism has long been an obstructor of the progress of knowledge in the field of touch, the corresponding attitude in connection with colour-phenomena has not been fatal to quite the same extent. It seems important, nevertheless, that we

---

[1] *Aufbau der Tastwelt*, p. 209.

consider that aspect of the visual sense with which we
are here concerned with respect to its dependence on
the temporal factor.   One immediate misunderstanding
must, however, be first dispelled.   Our concern here is
not with visual movement phenomena as movement
phenomena, for the psychology of perception of the last
few years is far from barren of such studies, but rather
with phenomena which come into being in connection
with movement without being identical with or charac-
terizable in terms of movement.   As an example I might
mention the phenomenon of the monocular stereoscopic
impression, whereby the suitable stimulation of *one* eye
over a particular time interval results in a highly plastic
impression, such as is normally produced only in binocular
vision.

We may take this example as our immediate point
of departure as we turn to those colour-phenomena which,
according to my observations, are directly dependent on
movement processes.   Now that we have seen how the
modes of appearance of colour are products of the union
of colour and space, it follows obviously that movement
must induce changes in all those colour-phenomena
which are dependent on spatial conditions which are
themselves subject to modification through movement.
In the foregoing passages I have already had occasion to
refer to such colour-phenomena.   Our concern here is
to review these phenomena once more from this different
theoretical point of view, and bring them into relationship
with other phenomena.

It has already been said that lustre is particularly
pronounced when movement is involved.   More specifically it must be noted here that lustre which appears in
connection with movement is strictly speaking not to be
identified with the lustrous appearance produced by a
stationary object, even when that object has been exposed
for a very brief interval.   When we see a lustrous point
shifting about on a moving object, all the successive
impressions—the not-yet-lustrous, the fully lustrous and
the subsequent no-longer-lustrous—belong together in a

single phase which, taken as a whole, represents an appearance fundamentally different from that of stationary lustre. Movement makes it possible for this impression to build itself up through a period of time, but it is unitary throughout. In this experience time itself, even the impression of movement, recedes completely. Just as I have described it in the case of touch experiences, which have been analogously built up, the movement is to a certain extent exhausted in the process of awakening another impression. In cases of sparkle and glitter the relationships are quite similar, and, as far as structure is concerned, even more obvious. In contrast to lustre, sparkle and glitter are never presented as stationary, but are always seen as moving. A sparkle is not to be considered summatively as the resultant of a great many tiny individual sparks, bound together in a single coherence-plane, nor is a glitter to be thought of as a combination of individually shining points. The assumption that in sparkle and glitter we have specific colour-experiences may be challenged—although it is not easy to do so. No one can, however, challenge the fact that sparkle and glitter are experiences which are built up in time and are produced by movement. Without movement they simply do not occur.

It has already been pointed out that the clearness of transparent impressions is enhanced by movement. One can assert further not only that transparency becomes clearer but even that it is to a certain extent a different kind of transparency. Without movement this kind of transparency is not to be found. The close relationship which obtains between transparency and the phenomenon of the coherence-plane makes it self-evident that all phenomena connected with the coherence-plane are clearer in movement than when in a state of rest. The connection between coherent particles receives, as it were, its primary confirmation through movement ; and the fact that the particles are not displaced during movement represents the primary guarantee of the stability of the coherence-plane. An exactly corresponding en-

hancement of clearness as a result of movement is to be
noted in connection with the phenomena of reflection
from colourless and coloured mirrors.

When we see a shadow or a light-spot drifting across
an object, we have the impression, not merely that the
shadow or light is standing out in clearer relief from the
ground, but also that the shadow or light has become an
existent *sui generis* in time. The stationary spot is like
an attenuated residue of the moving spot.

I have not striven here for completeness in my
description of those phenomena in the field of colour-
vision which owe their existence to movement. Further
and more specialized studies will have to be made, and
an eye that has been trained in the school of the motion
picture will probably have more success than an eye whose
education has been perverted by the microtomizing snap-
shots of bygone years.

§ 4. The Modes of Appearance in Everyday Language

The terms " surface colour," " film colour " and
" volume colour," which we have been employing, are
not to be found in everyday speech, and even when
presented as creations of an artificial psychological language they would not be readily understood without
further explanation. The remarks which we made above
about the relationship between the perceptual world and
the world of speech may not be extended without reservation to apply to artificial languages, but are rather to be
limited to languages which have developed naturally. It
is pertinent to ask the question whether or not differences
in mode of appearance of colour are in any way reflected
in linguistic expression. This is actually the case, even if
the material is not exactly abundant. I shall confine
myself to the reproduction of a few relevant findings,
culled from the afore-mentioned articles by Weisgerber.

Weisgerber in his discussion is not concerned with our
phenomenology of colour, but confines himself rather to

the setting up of two principal types of colour-perception
in contrast with each other, namely the phenomena of
lustre and all non-lustrous phenomena, which he designates
simply as " colour-phenomena." Thus it would appear
to us that objects on the one hand are blue, yellow, red,
etc., and on the other hand sparkle, shine, glitter, etc.
And there can be no doubt that because of this linguistic
peculiarity we have grown accustomed to seeing, in the
first case, properties of things, and, in the second case,
effects of those things on us or processes taking place on
them. From the phenomenological point of view we
have, it is true, to distinguish lustre, luminosity and
sparkle from each other. Weisgerber is, nevertheless,
thoroughly justified in recognizing an opposition between
stationary colour-phenomena, such as surface colours,
non-luminous film colours and volume colours, and all
those colour-phenomena, such as lustre, luminosity,
sparkle, flicker, and glitter, which either possess an inner
activity themselves or appear in connection with actual
movement. " Even if colour-phenomena [in Weisgerber's
sense] are in the main apprehended adjectivally, there are
nevertheless a few expressions in which they appear also
as verbs . . . a paper yellows with age . . . the sky
reddens, the day darkens. Thus we find three verbs . . .
which do not express as it were the coming into being
of a state, such as reddening (inchoative) . . . but which
simply render by verbs an expression which we would
otherwise apprehend adjectivally . . . the trees are green
and the trees turn green ; . . . in the latter case there is
a suggestion of the operation of a force which elicits the
green. . . . We have a counterpart in the field of lustre
in the form of a few adjectives. . . . This adjectival way
of apprehending phenomena of lustre is, however, quite
rare." Weisgerber has also traced certain changes from
the adjective to the verb characterization of colour-
impressions, discernible over a period of centuries. This
opens up an interesting field of investigation for psychologists, namely that of changes in modes of visual apprehension, such as, for example, the change toward the

c

impressionistic way of seeing, which reached its height about fifty years ago, and which has now in turn given way to something entirely different.

The colour-phenomena which owe their existence to movement stand close to the impressions of touch, not only with reference to their temporal aspects, but also, it is pertinent to point out here, with reference to ways in which they are characterized in language. " The stone is hard, the meadow is green, but the brook babbles, the thunder peals. . . . Thus auditory properties are expressed in the verb."[1]

§ 5. Non-Perceptual Colours

The foregoing analyses referred to modes of appearance of colours presented in perception. How do colours appear when they possess a non-perceptual character? The material that can be adduced in this connection is not very plentiful, largely because until now practically no attention has been paid to the question.

When visual hallucinations are strong, they seem to appear in non-transparent surface colours. This has to be assumed in all cases in which the hallucinated object completely covers what lies behind it. When the hallucinations are weaker, the hallucinated object appears transparent or translucent, either as somewhat filmy or as somewhat voluminous.[2] Pick describes hallucinations of a filmy character.[3] In eidetic images, which are closely related to hallucinations, distinct surface colours are possible.[4] Jaensch found that eidetic images of objects, as distinguished from eidetic images of pictures, tended to possess the character of surface colour. Sometimes the eidetic image seems to modify the mode of appearance of the ground against which it is seen. " The homogeneous background, seen simultaneously with the image, appears

[1] W. Haas, *Die psychische Dingwelt.* Bonn, 1921.
[2] Hartmann, *Monatschr. f. Psychiatr. u. Neurol.*, 1924, 56.
[3] A. Pick, *Neurol. Zentralblatt*, 1919, No. 20.
[4] O. Kroh, *Subjektive Anschauungsbilder bei Jugendlichen.* Göttingen, 1922.

to the eidetics not as the surface colour that it really is but rather as voluminous, cloudy or misty."[1]   Herwig and Jaensch, too, have like Kroh established the fact of transparency in eidetic images.[2]

Inasmuch as I have here anticipated certain observations to be discussed in detail in another context, I shall merely call attention to the fact that after-images of presented colours of any mode of appearance all have the tendency, when seen with closed eyes, to appear as film colours. If the original visual presentation is plastic, composed, for instance, of glowing filaments lying in different planes, a depth effect may be observable in the after-image as well.[3]   And if the after-image is projected outward, an impression of transparency may under suitable circumstances develop.[4] Weil claims to have observed lustre in after-images.[5]

The colours which appear in synæsthesias seem to possess a tendency to look filmy or voluminous.[6]

The visual images of normal non-eidetic people all tend more or less toward the filmy mode of appearance.[7] This holds, too, for the colours which appear in dream images. In my own dreams I have often been struck by an unusually strong appearance of luminosity. The colours found in the imagery induced by such drugs as mescal are also frequently described as luminous.

§ 6. How Other Sense-Impressions Appear

Parallel studies of modes of appearance in other fields have as yet been made only in connection with touch; in other sense modalities we have merely the beginnings of corresponding analyses. Quite early in my investigations I felt that if the problems connected with the modes

[1] A. Gösser, Zsch. f. Psychol., 1921, 87.
[2] B. Herwig and E. R. Jaensch, Zsch. f. Psychol., 1928, 87.
[3] R. Baruch, Zsch. f. Sinnesphysiol., 1928, 59.
[4] Fuchs, I, p. 201.   [5] H. Weil, Zsch. f. Psychol., 1929, 110.
[6] A. Argelander, Das Farbenhören und der synästhetische Faktor der Wahrnehmung. Jena, 1927.
[7] G. E. Müller, Zur Analyse der Gedächtnistätigkeit und des Vorstellungsverlaufes. Leipzig, 1911, p. 56 ff.

of appearance of sensory impressions were to become clear, analyses would have to be carried through in widely different sensory fields ; and my investigation of the sense of touch confirmed my expectation that such parallel studies would disclose valuable new points of view. We shall rapidly glance through those results from the touch study which are relevant to the present discussion.

In the field of touch, as in the field of colour, we can distinguish between two factors, touch matter and mode of appearance of touch matter. The analogy is fundamental, but in spite of this there is a noteworthy difference. In contrast to the wealth of colour-matter (black, white, red, yellow . . .) we have in touch matter an extraordinary monotony. " The polymorphism of the world of touch stands in striking contrast to the monotony of touch matter, for touch matter is moulded into a world of forms at least as rich and varied as the world of colour." [1] I have demonstrated the fact that corresponding to surface colour there is a surface touch, and corresponding to the pure unstructured visual quality of film colour there is a similar unstructured touch quality. Volume colours can be placed side by side with volume touches. And corresponding to transparent and translucent colours we have touch experiences of surfaces felt through other objects. Like the visually apprehended surface structure of surface colours, the surface structure which we apprehend tactually is of tremendous biological significance. And, finally, for Hering's memory colours there is a somewhat surprising parallel in the phenomena which I have characterized as memory touches.

In the field of touch there is nothing to correspond to illumination in the field of vision, and for this reason the world of touch lacks parallels for all those phenomena which in vision result from the interaction of colour and illumination. With respect to objectification and subjectification, the phenomena of touch and the phenomena of colour must be placed in different positions. Colour-phenomena are always characterized by objectification ;

[1] *Aufbau der Tastwelt*, p. 24.

they are always seen " out there " in space. This applies even to such phenomena as after-images or the intrinsic visual grey, which owe their existence solely to conditions in the retina or the visual cortex, and are quite independent of external objects. When we speak of subjective visual sensations we do so merely to indicate the absence of an objective stimulus source ; we never imply that they possess an immanent property which permits them to be experienced as belonging phenomenally to our own bodies. If we actually experience colour-phenomena as subjective, we do so only with the assistance of certain secondary cues. No matter how intently we project ourselves into a subjective phenomenon, such as that of the intrinsic visual grey, we can never succeed in catching even a faint trace of the feeling that it is something belonging to our own bodies. With touch phenomena, however, it is quite different. Here we have a combination, seemingly indissoluble, of two components, one subjective with a body reference, and the other objective, suggesting properties of objects. For this reason I have described touch phenomena as bi-polar. At one moment the subjective pole in a touch phenomenon may be dominant, and at another moment the objective pole, but this bi-polarity always persists. The same holds true for impressions of temperature. The very expressions we use when we talk about sensations sometimes reveal the distribution of accent. " When we formulate judgments about temperature we say sometimes, as we could in dealing with vision : ' It is warm, it is cold,' and sometimes, as we could never do in connection with vision : ' I am or I feel warm or cold.' " [1]

In the field of sound v. Hornbostel has called attention to certain differences in acoustic mode of appearance, and in some places he speaks directly of " modes of appearance of sound." [2] The severance of matter and mode of appearance is perhaps not as simple for tone as it is for

---

[1] U. Ebbecke, *Pflügers Arch.*, 1917, 169, p. 396.
[2] E. v. Hornbostel, *Handbuch d. norm. u. pathol. Physiol.*, 11. Berlin, 1926.

colours or touches, but when v. Hornbostel speaks of the
thickness and the sharpness of contour of a tone he is
probably referring to mode of appearance. We shall have
occasion later to speak of other striking contributions
made by v. Hornbostel. Further data bearing upon the
question as to how tone matter is presented are to be
found in a work by Werner.[1]

§ 7. ILLUMINATION AND EMPTY SPACE

One searches Hering's writings in vain for a statement
that the experience of illumination is an independent
factor in ordinary colour-perception. In the first edition
of this book I have, however, repeatedly called attention
to the phenomenal reality of illumination impressions.
One of the consequences of my interpretation of the way
in which illumination is presented has been that greater
weight than ever is now being laid upon the phenomenon
of illumination. There has developed, in fact, a doctrine
which holds to the primacy of illumination in normal
visual perception. I am in this connection in partial
agreement with certain views expressed by Bühler. In
a reply to my review of his work he writes : " How about
the factor of illumination when I have nothing before me
in the visual field but the blue sky, in other words nothing
but a pure film colour ? How about the factor of
illumination when I look into the blackened tube of a
spectroscope, and have nothing before me but the pure
film colour of a spectral field ? The colour that I see is
' luminous ' ; it seems to me that the phenomenon of
luminosity is closely connected with what we are accustomed to call the factor of illumination. How about the
illumination factor in an aperture field, when I cast
a visible shadow over both aperture and reduction
screen ? "[2] By contrasting my view with that expressed
here by Bühler I hope to be able to make clear what I
believe constitutes the essence of the phenomenon of

[1] H. Werner, *Grundfragen der Intensitätspsychologie.* Leipzig, 1922.
[2] K. Bühler, " Gegenbemerkungen," *Psychol. Forsch.*, 1925, 5, p. 187.

illumination. In a field like this, where our observation is phenomenological, it is particularly difficult to avoid slipping into a physical mode of thinking, and, if I make no mistake, Bühler has not quite succeeded in avoiding this danger. Physically speaking " illumination of something " and " light-source for something " are always connected. In the phenomenological sense, however, luminous colours and illumination factor are by no means inseparably united. The film colour appearing in a spectroscope is definitely luminous, and even when the intensity of the light used is increased somewhat it is still luminous, but it does not appear as illuminated, and illuminated objects do not necessarily appear in conjunction with it. Equally incorrect, it seems to me, would be the statement that the blue of the sky appears as illuminated. It can undoubtedly be luminous, but the factor of illumination is not given in it. The necessity for a sharp phenomenological distinction between luminosity and illumination can be very prettily demonstrated by means of an example, the strikingness of which impressed me even when I was a boy. If on a dark night we sally forth into the open with a red lantern, and hold this lantern above us in the direction of the open sky, we will then see a beautiful luminous red circle and around it pitch blackness. In such a case we need see no illumination, and there is none to see as long as the lantern does not by chance illumine some previously unseen objects. I remember that I was always disturbed by the apparent inability of the light of the lantern to produce an impression of illumination as long as the rays did not fall upon any objects. Such an observation shows how pronounced luminosity can be present without being accompanied by illumination. Such a lantern can be used, moreover, to demonstrate how an indubitable impression of illumination can be produced in the absence of any simultaneous luminosity in the visual field. If the lantern is so adjusted that it cannot itself be seen, but that its light is cast upon a number of objects, the result is a compelling impression of illumination, which is no less clear than if the lantern itself were seen at the same time. As a rule, when the lantern is concealed the illumination as such is even more clearly visible, because the observer is not blinded by the bright light. Later experiments will provide repeated confirmation of the fact that impressions of illumination are always quite independent of the perception of the light-sources, which, from a physical point of view, are involved in their production. It might be mentioned in this connection that, even when we represent illumination in pictures, it is quite unnecessary for us to paint in the light-source as well.

Another proof of the phenomenal independence of impressions of illumination and of luminosity, which we shall discuss in greater detail in another context, is to be found in the fact that in isolated eccentric portions of the retina we can have perfectly clear and convincing examples of luminosity, but we can never have impressions of illumination.

Under what conditions, then, can we have an impression of illumination ? May I suggest the following simple experiment. Close your eyes, and then open them for a very short time, just long enough to permit you to determine what kind of impression the visual field, as it is filled with objects of all sorts, makes upon you. Every-one will, I am sure, agree that at the moment at which the eyes are opened one has a fairly definite impression of a general illumination which seems to be dominant in the visual field. If, for instance, we compare under such conditions the relative difficulty of a judgment as to the colours in the visual field and a judgment as to its illumination, there can be no doubt that the latter is by far the easier. Care must be taken, however, that there be no initial set favouring either colour or illumina-tion. When the set is neutral, even the shortest opening of the eyes will permit some kind of report upon the colours of the objects seen in the central part of the visual field (although not upon the colours of peripherally distributed objects). It will always, however, be possible to report upon the dominant illumination. The impression of illumination forces itself immediately upon one, more so than do the colours of individual objects, unless brightness or saturation factors make the latter stand out unusually clearly from the background. The observation can be repeated with the eyes directed toward different parts of the room, and consequently toward differently coloured objects. Whatever the change in local colour may be, however, the impression of illumination is always present, and it always remains exactly the same. Such observations lead us to the conclusion that there is a non-derived, non-inferred primary impression of the illumination of the visual field, which from the point of view of experience is genetically prior to the experience of the individual colours of the objects which fill the visual field. This becomes particularly clear where the illumination is unusually strong or unusually weak. If we repeat the observations in the street in twilight, we find it exceedingly difficult to report upon the colours of houses and footpaths but quite easy to report upon illumination. It would be quite erroneous to say that the judgment of the illumination as weak was mediated by the observation that no secure judgment about colour could be made. On the contrary, the impression of illumination is perfectly immediate. Corresponding observations can be made with extremely intense illuminations at the seashore, for instance, at the noon hour on a bright midsummer day. If we open our eyes for a brief interval the impression of brilliant illumination is almost overpowering, but it is almost impossible to say anything about the colours of individual objects seen.

The foregoing observations do not apply to the extremes in the range of illumination. In a room from which all light has been excluded we have an absolute darkness, in which no objects can be seen. It would be descriptively incorrect to say that here we perceive a very weak illumination. We perceive in fact no illumination at all, but have rather the intrinsic visual grey which cannot be characterized in terms of illumination. If we allow direct sunlight to pass through closed eyelids, what we have is a luminous sea of light. We know theoretically, of course, that light is falling upon us, but with the disappearance of object perception the impression of illumination disappears too, and its place is taken by an impression of intense luminosity. What can we infer from this ? Our conclusion must be that a convincing impression of illumination can appear only where objects are apprehended, and that wherever objects are apprehended there must be an impression of illumination.

There can be no doubt that illumination is perceived with objects and by means of objects ; it is equally certain that illumination is perceived in the *empty space* which lies before objects. The word " empty " here must be stressed to distinguish it from space which is filled with fog or is otherwise beclouded. Space-filling media are a condition of the volume colours which we have already described in some detail. Volume colours, too, may help to determine the general impression of illumination ; we can see fog both in twilight and in full sunlight. Just at present, however, we are not interested in these phenomena, but rather in really empty space. Empty space appears in general as illuminated in the same way as do the objects which bound and delimit it. It is perhaps preferable to speak of a *lighting* of empty space, and thus to make the lighting of the empty space in the visual field correspond to the illumination of the objects in the visual field. I cannot characterize the relationship between empty space and light more adequately than by saying that empty space is filled with light (strong light, weak light, etc.). The relationship between illumination of objects and lighting of empty space may become more intelligible in the light of some further observations, which have the added merit of taking into account the case in which different parts of the visual field are differently illuminated at the same time. " If we stand before a wall, the illumination of which is essentially uniform (in the physical sense), we have no hesitation in attributing to the empty space in front of it a phenomenal character of brightness or of being filled with light (*Erleuchtung*), which is in keeping with the brightness of the wall, and is in a sense equal to it. If the intensity with which the objects are illuminated is changed uniformly, the lighting of the empty space changes in proportion. If the visual field is variously illuminated, in part normally, perhaps, and in part by direct sunlight, the illumination impression created by the whole empty space in front of the wall is determined by that part of the visual field the illumination of which is apprehended as dominant. Thus the space appears in normal illumination when all the objects, with the exception possibly of a few shadow-spots or light-spots, appear as normally illuminated. Immediately before the shadow-spots or light-spots, however, the space seems to assume the corresponding deviating brightness without at the same time presenting any clear-cut dividing line to indicate where one spatial brightness gives place to another. Similar relationships can be observed in a visual field in which the different parts are illuminated in qualitatively different ways."[1]

Differently illuminated objects can, strictly speaking, not lie one directly behind another, but are presented rather simply as touching one another or intercepting one another, so that illuminations of different kinds can be perceived only as side by side. Empty spaces, on the other hand, presenting different kinds of lighting, can be seen one behind another as well as side by side. "Let us look through the unlighted interior of a blackened tube, set up in a normally illuminated room in such a way that there is a space between the end of the tube and the farther wall of the room. We then see the space in front of the tube and beyond it in its normal brightness, but the space within the tube appears as clear—one is tempted to say luminous—darkness. This darkness has nothing in common with the misty darkness of a fog,

[1] D. Katz, Neue Beiträge zu den Erscheinungsweisen der Farben ; Luftlicht und Beleuchtungseindruck, *Zsch. f. Psychol.*, 1924, 95.

nor even with the dull darkness of the shadowed corner of a room. No sharp line can be drawn, it is true, between differently lighted spaces, but there always remains that remarkable phenomenon of empty spaces, lying one behind another, with clearly distinguishable, one might almost say mutually contrasting, brightnesses." Forsaking for the moment the purely descriptive approach, we may note in passing that the way in which empty space is lighted depends directly upon the mode of illumination of the objects which fill it and delimit it. When we consider the closeness of the connection between the impression of illumination presented by objects and the impression of lighting presented by the adjacent empty space, we may feel ourselves justified in speaking of them as co-variant phenomena.

It was probably the striking sensory clearness of the lighting of empty space which led Bühler to assume the light reflected by air particles as the stimulus basis for the perception of illumination. This assumption has not proved acceptable, but the indubitably sensory character of the impression of illumination, and the presupposition that for every factor in visual perception there must be a demonstrable objective stimulus, rendered it highly plausible. This latter presupposition will be discussed anew in the light of the totality theory of perception, which will later be brought to bear upon the problems of illumination and of space-lighting. It may, too, have been the strikingly sensory character of the lighting of empty space which, in the final analysis, determined Jaensch to set up his parallel laws of contrast and transformation ; for underlying this parallel lies the implicit assumption that the circumfield, " illuminated space," functions as *objective stimulus* affecting the infield, " illuminated colour," in exactly the same way as in ordinary surface contrast the objective stimulus of the circumfield affects the infield. This assumption is unjustified, for the air-light in such cases does not constitute an adequate light stimulus. Other objections to Jaensch's theory will be discussed later. Inasmuch, however, as we are here concerned with an understanding of its psychological basis, we may mention Jaensch's theory as evidence for the sensory character of the impression of illumination.   The perception of empty space filled with a medium differs somewhat from the perception of space filled with light, and for this reason the problem of spatial media deserves special consideration.[1]

The problem of spatial media was attacked by Jaensch. In his experiments he set up shadowed or illuminated corners, some of which were empty and some of which contained hanging threads.   " The impression of a coloured medium is present or absent, clear or lacking in pronouncedness, according as the attention is directed toward a point in the medium itself or toward one of the bounding surfaces."[2]   As I found in connection with transparent colours, Jaensch found that in the perception of a medium the adoption of an uncritical, natural attitude brings about an enhancement of clearness.   It is important, if we are to characterize Jaensch's medium in terms of our modes of appearance, to note that " an impression of depth does not necessarily involve the perception of a medium " (p. 275).   This observation, plus the reports of observers who, instead of seeing a spatial medium " looked right through " the air, would indicate quite clearly that spatial media must look very much like volume colours.   A few of Jaensch's remarks might be understood as implying that empty space is given only when it is filled with a spatial medium.   This view, however, seems to me untenable, and in fact tends to contradict certain other statements made by Jaensch. We have already described cases of volume colour in which indubitable space-filling media in Jaensch's sense are present.   To these may be added the phenomena of twilight vision and the cases in which parts of the visual field appear as clearly shadowed.   In some of the latter

[1] Cf. A. Gelb, " Die Farbenkonstanz der Sehdinge," *Handbuch d. normal. u. pathol. Physiol.*, 12.   Berlin, 1929, p. 634 ff.   Hereafter cited as Gelb.
[2] E. R. Jaensch, *Die Raumwahrnehmung des Auges.*   Leipzig, 1911, p. 259 f.

there is no trace of a space-filling medium of any kind. Jaensch's descriptive report of the relationship between space-filling media and volume colours can, it seems to me, be confirmed in many cases. With his theory of space-filling media, however, I cannot agree.[1] Assuming, then, that Jaensch's space-filling medium can be located fairly clearly in the scheme of modes of appearance of colour, it must be clear, too, that the experience of truly empty space must be thought of in terms other than those of space-filling media. An empty space, which does not in any way becloud the things behind it, is given as strongly or weakly or as chromatically or achromatically lighted. I am implying no psychological *horror vacui* when I formulate the proposition that empty space can be given only in such a way that it appears as filled with chromatic or achromatic light of varying intensity.

Extensive studies of the ways in which empty space is presented have been made by Schumann.[2] According to him empty space is given sensorially in the form of a special sensation, which he terms the " glassy " sensation. This is supposed to be particularly easy to observe when one looks at pictures through a stereoscope, but less clear under the ordinary conditions of vision on a bright day. In our attempt to decide how empty space is usually given, however, it is perhaps best not to lay too much weight on the results of stereoscopic observations,

---

[1] D. Katz, *Zur Psychologie des Amputierten und seiner Prothese*. Leipzig, 1921. According to Jaensch persistent central excitation in the visual sector constitutes the physiological basis of perceived space-filling media. He accepts, in this connection, Holt's view (*Psychol. Rev. Mon. Suppl.*, 1903, 4) that, as long as the central processes underlying eye-movement are in operation, retinal impressions are transmitted to consciousness either not at all or in greatly reduced intensity. There are some observations which make it seem probable to me that the central processes underlying eye-movement do have an anæsthetic effect in the sense that the recognition of objects becomes impossible. They do not, however, prevent retinal excitation from having an effect on consciousness. If we close our eyes, and allow light to pass through the lids, we will have light sensations in keeping with the nature and intensity of the light. Now with a little practice it is possible to keep our eyeballs continuously rolling. During such eye-movements the original visual sensation remains essentially unchanged. Thus we have no right to speak of a total central anæsthesia during eye-movement.

[2] F. Schumann, *Zsch. f. Psychol.*, 1920, 85.

for here, as v. Frey has pointed out,[1] the very technical incompleteness of the presented pictures may produce an unnatural effect. Stereoscopic observations, too, have revealed the fact that under such conditions space appears as filled with fine dust, and the duller the paper chosen for the photograph the clearer this impression is. The texture of the paper affects disparate retinal points, and in this way produces the impression that the space before the picture is filled with dust.

Both the strength and the quality of perceived illumination are in large measure determined by the objective intensity and colour of the illumination dominant in the visual field. During the course of the day the intensity of the illumination, and therewith the impression of illumination, usually increases steadily until the sun has reached its greatest height, and then gradually declines until finally twilight sets in. Even if we confine ourselves to those illuminations which involve primarily cone vision, we have still a tremendous range of distinguishable impressions of illumination. As long as the whole visual field is illuminated with approximately equal intensity we may speak of a uniform illumination. Perfectly uniform illumination, of course, could hardly occur under ordinary circumstances, for when an object is seen in even vague relief the effect is usually due to the fact that its different parts are differently illuminated. In such cases the dominant illumination is broken by shadows and superimposed lights, and these in themselves merit separate consideration. I shall follow the lead here of Bühler, who has accepted Leonardo da Vinci's classification of shadows into conjoined shadows, air shadows and cast shadows.

"Wherever light from one direction falls upon an opaque object, *e.g.*, a ball, the opposite side remains unilluminated, *i.e.*, shadowed; and this shadow clings to the shadow-casting object. Beyond it the shadow-cone passes through the air until it is caught by a new surface

---

[1] M. v. Frey, *Zsch. f. Biol.*, 1921, 73. *Cf.* also E. F. Möller, "The Glassy Sensation," *Amer. J. Psychol.*, 1925, 36.

and extends itself like a membrane over this surface (cast shadow).[1] Conjoined shadows are of importance primarily inasmuch as they are responsible for the plastic appearance of objects ; the conjoined shadow is the real modeller of the object. A ball can be illuminated and set up before a background in such a way that its cast shadow is not visible without at the same time having any of its plastic character sacrificed. The conjoined shadow, as the very name suggests, clings so closely to the surface of its object that it is practically impossible to see it as distinct from the genuine colour of the object. An air-shadow causes the empty space in which it is seen to appear darker, and it appears as a medium filling this space, whereas the spaces before and behind it are seen as distinctly brighter. The situation here is similar to that which we observed in connection with differently lighted spaces lying one behind another. When we turn to cast shadows we find that in general the deeper the cast shadow the more it eats its way into the colour of the object, and the weaker it is the more readily it tends to assume the character of a " shadow membrane " (Bühler). When it is in motion it seems to belong least of all to the surface of the object. " There are some very weak degrees of shadow and boundaries of shadow which can be perceived only when they are in motion, and which are otherwise quite invisible, even when we know exactly where they are." [2] I might add that according to my own observation a shadow which has begun to move becomes darker, but at the same time induces a smaller change in the colour of the surface across which it is moving. When a shadow moves it moves not *in* the surface of the object but *across* it. Here we have one of the afore-mentioned cases in which movement in time serves to call into being an entirely new type of colour-phenomenon. A colour which moves across another colour, without at the same time inducing any change in it, is a strikingly new phenomenon. Bühler is correct when he says that the painter, in representing shadow,

---

[1] Bühler; p. 76.   [2] *Ibid.*, p. 77.

has no way of picturing " the shifting and drifting of shadows over objects, and *vice versa* the slipping by of objects under a stationary shadow." " If you attempt to brush a small shadow which looks like a spot of dirt from the arm of your coat, a slight arm movement is quite sufficient to restore your peace of mind by changing it into its proper mode of appearance."[1]

For the perception of moving cast shadows there is an optimal speed, above and below which the shadow has to be deeper to be equally perceptible. Thus change of position and change in depth of shadow have opposite effects. A change of the latter kind, which must, of course, be artificially induced, does not make the shadow stand out more clearly, but tends rather to fuse it more completely with the colour of the surface. Other conditions being held constant, the stronger the configuration of a shadow the less it stands out in its own right. As a rule, cast shadows appear most convincingly on surfaces. I have, however, observed them occasionally on volume colour, *e.g.*, on clouds of mist. An air-shadow is never seen as an extended membrane, but tends rather to reduce the lighting of the space in which it is seen and fill it with darkness. Thus the perfect clarity of empty space is replaced by a space-filling medium. The fact that a shadow cast upon a surface is not seen simply as a local reduction in brightness, as though a paint-brush had been applied, is due to the preservation of the microstructure of the surface. The miscrostructure continues to be seen " undimmed and undistorted beneath the shadow membrane."[2]

One of Hering's classical experiments with shadow has proved extraordinarily fruitful. " If I suspend a bit of paper from a thread before a lamp in such a way that a faint shadow is cast upon my writing-pad, I see the shadow then as a casual dark spot lying on the white of the paper. If, however, I now draw a broad black line about the shadow, so as to cover the penumbra completely, what I see within the black line is a grey spot, which

---

[1] Bühler, p. 80.   [2] *Ibid*, p. 80.

D

looks exactly as if the white paper had been coloured with grey paint or a grey paper with a black border had been pasted on the white."[1] Bühler has pointed out that the decisive factor in the destruction of the shadow impression cannot be the annihilation of the penumbra by the black line, for even a black line drawn *through* the shadow can destroy the impression of shadow in the adjacent areas and make the darkness look like colour. The line removes the depth severance, and fuses the darkness of the shadow into the colour of the paper.

The phenomenal opposite of a shadow-spot is a super-imposed light-spot. Here again we may quote from Hering. "A beam of sunlight passes through a hole in the window-shutter, and falls upon a limited portion of my black coat; I see a grey spot there, and try to brush it off. As soon, however, as I observe the place somewhat more closely, I see that it is no longer a spot of dust, but merely a ray of light falling upon the black of the coat, and now, even in indirect vision, I can scarcely restore the original impression. Or I pass along a heavily shadowed pathway in the forest, and a single ray of light breaks through the leafy covering and illumines a small portion of the path; for a moment I think that the whiteness I see is that of a pile of chalk; as soon as I observe more closely, however, I can see no more white, but merely light lying on the grey-brown earth."[2] In general all that we have said about shadows holds true for superimposed lights, although Bühler mentions a few differences between shadow-spots and light-spots. " Strong lights, *e.g.*, spots of sunlight, do not look like transparent membranes, and the painter does not use a transparent paint, like varnish, but uses rather an opaque white."[3] Space-filling media are to be seen in brightly lighted corners just as in shadowed corners, however, and movement has the same effect upon superimposed lights as it has upon shadows.

It follows from the foregoing that there is no hard and fast dividing line between impressions of generally reduced

---

[1] Hering, V, p. 8.   [2] *Ibid.*, p. 8 f.   [3] Bühler, p. 82.

or heightened illumination and impressions of shadow or superimposed light. The one impression gives way readily to the other when one approaches or withdraws from a complex of objects. If on a sunny day one stands immediately in front of the " shadowed " wall of a house, one sees no shadow but sees the wall and the space in front of it rather as well illuminated. But if one withdraws from the wall until it occupies but a small part of the visual field, and the rest of the field is in sunshine, the impression now is that the wall is in deep shadow and that the space in front of it is filled with a dark medium. Between these two limiting cases all possible intermediate stages can be observed. The greater the distance the more condensed the space-filling medium, the smaller the distance the more the medium tends to disappear and give place to a glassy empty space. A parallel series of stages can be observed when one withdraws from a strongly illuminated wall, which stands in the middle of a normally illuminated visual field. It is almost as though in the one case there were a certain quantum of darkness, and in the other a certain quantum of light, which have to be distributed through a particular space. The brighter the space before the wall appears, as the distance from it is increased, the darker the wall itself must appear, and the darker the intermediate space the brighter the wall. This reciprocal relationship between space brightness and object brightness (it holds *mutatis mutandis* also for chromatic illumination) is further illustrated by observations made by Jaensch when he set up his parallel laws of contrast and transformation.

§ 8. Colour-Matter and Mode of Appearance

If we think of all the film colours we ever experience as arranged in order, the result is the system of film colours. In the same way we can think together into a system the colours of another mode of appearance. Of all such systems that of the surface colours is by far the most significant for the studies which are to follow. Colours which belong to *different* systems may be termed *hetero-geneous*, as distinct from *homogeneous* colours which belong to the *same* system. In classifying colours it is customary to do so on the basis of the abstract attributes of hue, saturation and brightness. These attributes, which are found in every colour-impression quite apart from its particular mode of appearance, may be considered as indicating the "value" or "matter" of the colour. Heterogeneous colour-impressions may be equivalent in some or in all of the dimensions of "colour-matter."[1] Wherever in the present work we speak of an equality between two colour-impressions of differing mode of appearance, this implies merely that the impressions are equivalent in all the dimensions of colour-matter. As far as I can see there are practically no reports in the literature of experiments in which the attempt has been made to equate heterogeneous colour-impressions. It would appear that Hering's judgment of the impossibility of such equations has been tacitly accepted. "A per-fectly satisfying equation between two colours is possible," he writes, "only when the external conditions, which, apart from the nature and intensity of the light stimuli and the sensitivity of the relevant parts of the visual apparatus, can have an influence on perception, are, if not excluded, at least exactly the same for both colours. Thus, apart from the fact that they are side by side, both colours should be localized in exactly the same way, and each should be so perfectly homogeneous that it presents no irregularities and appears, not as belonging to some specific external object, but rather as an independently existent plane or space-filling *quale*."[2] Hering's dictum is probably warranted as a principle to be followed in the study of the psychological effects of different physical wave-lengths. In so far, however, as Hering would limit all comparative studies of colour to film colours

---

[1] "Space is not an essential dimension of colour, but of mode of appearance of colour." K. Haack, *Experimental-deskriptive Psychologie der Bewegungen, Konfigurationen und Farben unter Verwendung des Flimmerphänomens.* Berlin, 1927, p. 253.
[2] Hering, VI, p. 12.

(and this is the logical implication of his dictum), the psychologist cannot accept his point of view. Hering insists in the foregoing quotation upon the importance of an equivalence of secondary conditions for a satisfactory equation between two colours. The expression " secondary conditions," however, covers a number of different factors which influence the appearance of a colour ; these might more profitably be kept distinct. Hering undoubtedly has the different modes of appearance in mind. It must be granted, too, that an equality between colours differing in mode of appearance is quite difficult to achieve. We find this, for instance, when we attempt to equate the hue of a paper (surface colour) with the hue of a spectral colour (film colour). It helps us very little in such a case to have the colours equal in size and shape, at the same distance and against the same background. I have found, in fact, that, even when we are dealing with colours of the same mode of appearance, differences in size, shape, distance and background do not make the equation much more difficult. If, for instance, two colour-wheels are presented against the same background, but at considerably different distances from the eye, it is not hard to find an equation between them for any single dimension of colour.

The literature contains an increasing number of reports to the effect that differences in mode of appearance can create difficulties in the equation of colours, a fact which has hitherto been generally overlooked. This has been noted, for instance, by Mintz,[1] by Benary [2] and by Ackermann.[3] It sometimes happens, too, that differences in mode of appearance may actually result in different settings when colours are equated. Two examples may be mentioned in illustration. Langfeld [4] found that when colours were being equated for brightness a change in the attitude of the observer might change his perception in such a way as to produce a quite different brightness equation for the same colour. A similar observation, too,

[1] A. Mintz, *Psychol. Forsch.*, 1928, 10, p. 314 f.
[2] W. Benary, *Psychol. Forsch.*, 1924, 5, p. 142.
[3] A. Ackermann, *Psychol. Forsch.*, 1924, 5.
[4] H. S. Langfeld, *Zsch. f. Psychol.*, 1909, 53.

was made by Matthaei.[1] He found that the same colour could have two brightnesses. When the observer was set for luminosity, with hue abstracted, the equation was brighter; when he was set for hue, with luminosity abstracted, the equation was darker. A set for density (in episcotister experiments; cf. § 45) yielded brighter values, and a set for transparency darker values.

Hitherto psychological textbooks have persistently over-looked mode of appearance in connection with the classification of colours. It is customary to speak simply of *colours*, and to assert that they vary in three dimensions, and that these dimensions can be illustrated by means of solid figures. "The colour-pyramid affords a clear, and at the same time, as the mathematicians put it, a *conformal mapping* of all possible variations within the world of colour."[2] The question one naturally asks, however, is: Of what mode of appearance are the colours upon which this scheme has been based? In the traditional colour-experiments, spectral colours and coloured papers have been used. Since these are film and surface colours, one suspects at once that it is film colours or surface colours which Ebbinghaus's scheme represents. Furthermore, the general tendency in the discussion of colour to abstract the factor of mode of appearance, *i.e.*, to consider it simply as film colour, makes it even more probable that when Ebbinghaus and others speak of sheer colour as such they are referring to film colour. As far as surface colours are concerned, at any rate, no adequate schematic representation has ever yet been devised.

We may, however, beg the question as to what type of colour has been employed in the earlier studies. Mode of appearance can be ignored as long as colours of the same mode of appearance are used for comparison. For this reason all existing colour-laws retain their validity, since they refer to what we have defined as "colour-matter." It is important that this point be explicitly

[1] R. Matthaei, *Zsch. f. Sinnesphysiol.*, 1928, 59.
[2] H. Ebbinghaus, *Grundzüge der Psychologie*, Vol. I, 2nd ed. Leipzig, 1905, p. 200.

recognized. The present investigation is concerned with aspects of colour which have not yet been dealt with. One problem is that of examining the relationship between colours of different modes of appearance, and toward this end a method which we may term the *method of reduction* has proved the most satisfactory. This method will be described in the next paragraph.

§ 9. THE REDUCTION OF COLOURS

What are the retinal processes underlying heterogeneous colours ? Have we any right to assume that there are retinal differences corresponding to differences in mode of appearance ? The following observations may help to answer these questions. Mention has already been made of the fact that an impression of surface colour can be changed to that of film colour with the assistance of an aperture screen. Even if the illumination of the surface colour deviates in any way from the " norm," so that it might be described as " not normally illuminated,"[1] it is still possible to transmute it into film colour with the aid of an aperture screen. In the same way the *voluminous* character of a colour can be replaced by that of film, and we have already noted specifically that lustre can be made to assume the film-colour appearance. The same holds true for colours of all other modes of appearance. We can always achieve this result by interposing a single or double aperture screen at a proper distance between the eye and that which is to be observed. This process we may term the *reduction of colour-impressions to the same mode of appearance.* The reduction of all colour-impressions to film colour is not a new discovery ; it is new, however, as a methodological principle for the comparative study of heterogeneous colours. The direction of this reduction process is always toward the film-colour appearance, never toward that of surface colour, volume colour, etc. This does not imply, however, that comparisons of different modes of appearance cannot be

[1] Cf. § 16.

made except in terms of film colour. Reduction to film colour merely affords us a practical way of comparing directly the retinal excitations corresponding to colours which look different. If this is really to be achieved, of course, precautions must be taken that the actual light stimulating the retina undergo no change *as a result of* the process of reduction. The excitation of a particular point on the retina is dependent on the state of the retina itself, on the wave-length and intensity of the light affecting it and on the surrounding light. Consequently, if we are to assert that retinal excitation has not been changed by the reduction process, we have to be sure that these factors have remained constant. Both before and after reduction the state of the retina must be exactly the same during observation. This condition can readily be fulfilled if both colour and illumination of the aperture screen are properly controlled. In the experiments to be reported it may always be assumed that these precautions have been taken. For the immediate purpose of the reduction process, namely that of rendering possible a comparison between the retinal excitations corresponding to colours of differing mode of appearance, it is not important to decide whether or not the illumination of the reduction screen exercises an influence on the reduced colour. Such an influence exists, as a matter of fact, but it will be discussed in another connection (§ 18). One of the essential facts about the reduction of colour is that it usually involves a change in its localization and a change in the way in which it fills space. After reduction the colour (the film colour) always appears at an indefinite distance behind the aperture screen. It is only in unusual cases that the accommodation of the observer's eye remains the same after reduction as before. In view of this change in accommodation, it might be suggested that reduction must then involve a physical change in the receptorial process, which would affect the intensity of retinal excitation. This, however, is not the case as long as the aperture in the screen remains completely and uniformly filled with the same light. Helmholtz has made this clear in his discussion of light intensity and diffusion circles on the retina.[1] Changes in intensity of retinal image, such as might be brought about by pupillary changes induced by shifts in accommodation, may be ignored as long as the reducing screen is kept at a given distance (more than 1 m.) from the observer's eye.[2] Under such conditions retinal excitation is independent of accommodation. What, then, do we learn from the use of the reduction screen ? The fact of most immediate importance is that different modes of appearance of the same colour are all based on the same retinal processes. Another way of stating it would be as follows : There is no colour-impression which *after* reduction is not exactly equal to a corresponding member of the film-colour system. Such a finding might be considered trivial, because as a matter of fact it is implicitly assumed in most studies of colour. The importance of its explicit formulation will, however, become clear in the light of the discussion to follow.

[1] Helmholtz, II, p. 113.
[2] Cf. Bach, *Pupillenlehre*. Berlin, 1908, p. 60.

PART II

FILM COLOURS

§ 10. The Subjective Visual Grey

The experiments upon subjective visual grey which I have performed leave no doubt about the fact that there are great individual differences in its mode of appearance.[1]

All observers agree that subjective visual grey is less definitely localized than any other colour. It lies, of course, in front of the eyes, but it is difficult to make a more definite report about its localization. I used the following method to train my observer. I brought an intensely luminous light-source before his closed eyes; now, when I removed quickly a piece of cardboard, which had been placed between the light-source and his eyes, so much light passed through his eyelids that a considerable brightening of the visual field could be observed. Even a person who can at first make no report about the localization of his subjective visual grey does not hesitate in his judgment concerning the approximate location of the observed change in light, nor, after some practice, in his judgment about the location of the subjective grey itself. The light which excites the retina, and which greatly exceeds the subjective grey in insistence, has the effect of turning attention in an unusual direction. In this case, not only the great intensity of the stimulus but also the change of light is itself a determiner of attention, since its effect is similar to that of movement in the visual field when the eyes are open. The observers

---

[1] " The field of after-images when the eyes are closed, or the black visual field, appears to me to be of very limited size, without any depth, and immediately before my eyes or coinciding with their vertical plane." G. T. Fechner, *Elemente der Psychophysik*. 2. Aufl. Leipzig, 1889. Teil II, p. 472.

report that the *change* of light is more definitely localized than the constant brighter light. After these drill-experiments were completed, we obtained the following reports on subjective grey. The centre of the grey or black field is localized by the various observers at a distance of approximately 10–40 cm.[1] I say the "centre," because for most observers the subjective grey does not seem to lie in one plane, and hence the various parts of its curved surface appear at different distances.

The surface in which the visual grey is presented seems, as a rule, to have a curvature concave toward the observer, a curvature described by many observers as "funnel-shaped." Even after all after-images have vanished, the subjective grey seldom has the same colour throughout. Sometimes its peripheral parts, at other times its central parts, seem distinctly brighter. The following report indicates that certain points of the visual field may be especially favoured by distribution of attention. "The whole thing has perhaps the form of a cone whose apex is the fixation-point and lies farthest away." We may make the following statements about the spatial organization of subjective grey. "The perception is comparable to a thick stratum of fog, through which we see no objects, or to a very turbid liquid, such as muddy water. The distance between this layer and the observer (perhaps 30 cm.), unlike the space between objects and the observer in twilight vision, is not filled distinctly with tri-dimensional darkness. The character of the perception of distance is comparable rather to the perception of the distance between objects and the observer in daylight illumination."[2] It is interesting to note that one observer

---

[1] Metzger has used a pretty procedure to determine these limits for his observers. "When a person is speaking with someone in complete darkness, the voice of the one who answers usually sounds distinctly *behind* the darkness, not in the darkness. . . . A measuring scale is extended to a point under the eyes of the observer, and the experimenter, talking continuously, moves slowly toward the observer until the latter reports that the speaker is *within* the dark wall." W. Metzger, *Psychol. Forsch.*, 1929, 13, p. 15. Hereafter cited as Metzger, I.

[2] Metzger, I, p. 9, adopts this description literally to characterize the impression which we get when the whole visual field is uniform but weakly illuminated.

likened his subjective grey to dark velvet, presumably to indicate a certain thickness in its layer of colour. We may add, by way of negative definition, that the subjective grey is not in the least related to surface colour. There is something voluminous about it, although it does not distinctly fill space in the tri-dimensional way to which we are accustomed in the case of strictly voluminous colours, such as a fog. We may say in summary : Aside from its individual peculiarities in mode of appearance, subjective grey has the mode of appearance of film colour, is related to volume colour and is very indefinitely localized.

According to well-grounded views, subjective grey has as its cause an endogenous excitation of the visual cortex.[1] We might suspect, therefore, that it would undergo no change unless the existing endogenous excitation were to be modified by a peripheral excitation. This supposition is not, however, justified. Some observers even report a change if they allow their eyes, while closed, to converge upon an imaginary point close before the face. In such cases the subjective grey seems to approach the observer and its area to decrease in extent. At the same time, however, the grey assumes a more stable structure, manifesting a certain condensation. I instructed the observers alternately to open and to close their eyes in a completely darkened room, and to determine whether they could perceive any change in their subjective grey. The reports of most of the observers indicate, partly directly and partly more indirectly, that when they open their eyes, the subjective grey becomes somewhat more definitely localized, and at the same time appears to move to a greater distance, while the plane in which it appears increases in extent.

Standing with open eyes in a darkened room, the observers looked to the left, to the right, upward and downward. The most noticeable change was in the form of a plane in which the subjective grey lay. Sometimes this bulged out in the direction toward which the eyes

[1] Müller, II, p. 40 ff.

had moved. The entire visual field also seemed at times to be moving toward the side in question. Finally, it is not without interest that, with circular turning of the head, many observers had the impression " that the field then observed was larger than before." While the subjective grey underwent changes in mode of appearance, no changes in brightness were observed in our experiment.[1]

We may say in summary that the mode of appearance of the subjective grey depends upon various attitudes, in spite of its endogenous origin. It is easy to see in the subjective grey a colour which, in certain respects, has the most " primitive " mode of appearance. It is, in any case, the colour with least figural character.

The Experiment with the Luminous Line.—In a completely darkened room I held before my open eyes a short, weakly luminous strip covered with luminous paint (hereafter called the luminous line), sometimes at a short distance (about 15 cm.) and at other times at a greater distance (about 1·5 m.). In spite of its minimal brightness, the luminous line exercises an interesting transforming process upon the field of the subjective grey. When it lies at the shorter distance (Case I), all observers note it as a rather definitely localized line standing out from the rest of the visual field. The immediate neighbourhood of the line, perhaps as broad as the line itself, appears deep black (as a result of simultaneous contrast), while the outlying surroundings recede distinctly. We observe quite a different transformation when the luminous line lies at a greater distance (Case II). It is then usually seen " as if it were on a small pillow," the grey extending distinctly *toward the observer*, so that he has the impression that the luminous line is placed in a funnel-shaped cavity.

I think that we may conclude with some certainty

---

[1] Observations of a blackening of the subjective grey with accommodation and convergence for near vision, as reported by E. R. Jaensch (*Zentralblatt f. Physiol.*, 1910, 24, p. 2 f.), were not reported spontaneously by my observers. It is an obvious assumption that the thickening of the colour-masses of the subjective grey, as mentioned above, was taken to be a blackening.

from these observations that when the position of the closed eyes is not disturbed, the grey lies at a distance *between* the two positions of the luminous line. The film of the normal subjective grey has, it is true, a certain concavity for almost all observers, but the normal bulging does not resemble in the least the funnel-shaped cavity observed here. The fact that the central portions of the grey film do not ordinarily lie at the distance of the luminous line in Case I seems to imply that in this case the observed film is convex. This deduction presupposes that the various parts of the grey tend to remain unchanged, in their normal mode of appearance, in the face of the transforming effect to which they are subjected by an impression localized at a definite distance ; and that a concavity or convexity of the visual field will obtrude more strongly (when the luminous line is used) the farther its new structure departs from the normal.[1]

§ 11. The Localization of Film Colours : Rôle of Colour-Matter and Configuration

When the closed eyes are illuminated directly, we perceive a brilliant orange, greatly exceeding the subjective grey both in brightness and in insistence. If we illuminate the closed eyes for a longer time in the way described, and then suddenly cover the light-source, we see, as a result of the after-image, greenish-blue colours which are considerably darker than the subjective grey.

---

[1] When isolated visual stimuli are introduced, space undergoes an expansion ; when they are removed, a contraction. Metzger has, with justice, pointed out that this contraction is reminiscent of the shortening of phantom-limbs, as I have described it, in patients whose limbs have been amputated, and that my views about the central processes regulating the behaviour of the phantom-limbs may be carried over, in their essential points, to relationships in visual space. " As regards the changes observed in the phantom-limb, we gain the impression that the limb is usually preserving its natural size and distance under the influence of special tensions. One may think of an elastic gas-filled balloon which retains its tension as long as the gas pressure continues undiminished, but begins to shrivel as soon as the gas pressure is reduced. In our case, the elastic balloon is represented by the surface of the limb, and the tensions arise from the manifold tactile, kinæsthetic and other impressions from the limb." D. Katz, *Psychologie des Amputierten und seiner Prothese.*, p. 38.

Neither the brighter nor the darker of these colours is as uniform as the subjective grey. The brighter colour seems, rather, to be relatively dark at its margin and the darker to be relatively bright in that region. According to observers' reports, the two colours are not as in-definitely localized as the subjective grey. We must, accordingly, distinguish various *degrees of indefiniteness of localization* even in the case of film colours. Usually the brighter colour lies at a greater distance than the subjective grey; also it appears more voluminous and, when the light-source is very intense, luminous. As for the perception of the darker colour, different observers agree that the space between them and the colour is experienced more distinctly than in the case of the grey; the darker colour itself, which like the brighter usually appears farther away than the grey, is less voluminous than the grey.

The difference between the localization of the grey and that of the brighter and darker colours produced during or after radiation of the closed eyes cannot be explained by any of the factors otherwise determining the localization of colour-impressions, either by a "primary" factor or by an empirical determinant in the traditional sense. We might explain the more definite localization when the retina is excited by the fact that the peripheral excitation produces a colour exceeding the subjective grey in insistence. The experiments reported below support this explanation.

There is no dearth of exhaustive studies of the localization of negative after-images projected upon the surfaces of objects. Other experiments have dealt fairly thoroughly with the distance of after-images when the eyes are closed, with special consideration of the question of the dependence of this distance upon the composition of the stimulus producing the after-image, as well as upon the convergence of the eyes. We do, however, lack observations dealing particularly with the question of the localization of the after-image in relation *to the background* upon which it appears when the eyes are closed. Whenever the after-image is projected upon an object having the mode of appearance of a surface colour, the question of its localization in relation to the background is easily answered. The after-image itself appears in the plane of the object, adapting itself to it in every irregularity and, as regards size, following Emmert's law. When the eyes are moved slowly, the after-image slips as a brighter or darker spot along the surface of the object, much as an objective moving spot of light or a shadow slips over it. I carried out two series of experiments to determine the localization of after-images with the eyes closed. Here I varied the spatial distribution of retinal excitation, its figural character, and the difference in hue and brightness between after-image and ground. The second series consists of observations in which the after-image was projected upon the sky, which is a pronounced film colour.

We have reported certain experiments in which the entire visual field was lightened or darkened. A simple variation of these experiments is to stimulate one half of the retina uniformly by a certain light, the other half equally uniformly by a different light. I laid side by side two rectangular papers large enough to fill the entire visual field and differing from each other in brightness or hue. (The following combinations were used : white-black, white-grey, black-grey, white with eight chromatic colours, and black with eight chromatic colours.) By fixating the middle of the boundary-line of the two papers, we produced two negative after-images of the original colours, and observed them with the eyes closed.

All the observers reported that they hardly ever had the positive impression that the after-images lay in one plane. There is, nevertheless, no simple relationship between differences in brightness or in hue and the localization of the after-images. It appears rather that when any two after-images are seen, the more insistent always tends to appear as nearer. There is considerable evidence that the impression of a displacement of the masses of colour in the visual field, or of two fields different in size, appears only as a result of a difference in insistence.

Is this relationship between the insistence and the distance of a colour partially dependent upon individual experience in everyday life ; or have we here an original interconnection which is, perhaps, present in the consciousness of a very young child ? There is much evidence favouring an original, unlearned interconnection between colours of certain insistences and certain depth-values. Our experience shows us that colours of extremely different brightnesses may lie in the same plane of an object. I have not found any decisive data in the case of congenitally blind who have recovered their vision.

In the following experiments a small part of the retina was subjected to special stimulation, so that instead of having the visual field divided into two equal parts, we had now a figural element present. To produce the after-images I used chromatic or achromatic paper circles pasted upon achromatic cardboard. In this way I was able to get approximately achromatic and distinctly chromatic after-images upon a lighter or darker achromatic background, so that all the more important cases of differences in colour and brightness between after-image and ground might be observed. The circles had a diameter of about 2·5 cm., and were observed from a convenient distance. The relationships in localization which we were investigating proved to be independent of this distance. It makes no difference in this connection whether the after-images are produced monocularly or binocularly.

Observation of negative after-images with the eyes closed leads to the generalization that after-images are almost always localized distinctly at a distance different from that of the ground. As regards the localization of the after-image *before* or *behind* the ground, we note the following tendencies : 1. A brighter chromatic or achromatic after-image always lies before a darker achromatic background. 2. A distinctly chromatic after-image always lies before an achromatic background whenever the latter is not much brighter than the after-image. 3. If an achromatic or chromatic after-image is considerably darker than an achromatic ground, there is in most cases an immediate impression that the after-image lies at a greater distance than the ground. The observers believe that they are then perceiving in the background an aperture through which they are looking at a dark disc. In this case, however, the observers can, with a certain effort, see a dark after-image lying in front of a brighter ground ; this impression appears spontaneously only in rare cases.

Let us summarize the results of these observations of after-images. If we eliminate those primary influences (accommodation, convergence, disparity of retinal images) which ordinarily determine the localization of coloured surfaces, and the " empirical "[1] determinants in the traditional sense, different excitation of different retinal points brings about a different localization of the resulting colour-sensations. Those colour-sensations which are distinguished, through their greater brightness, from a darker visual field or, through hue, from an achromatic field, are localized nearer than the rest of the visual field. Those which closely resemble in brightness the rest of the visual field are, in most cases, localized at a greater distance than the rest of the field ; sometimes, however, they may be localized nearer.

What, then, is the mode of appearance of after-images as we see them with closed eyes ? They appear as film colours. This does not mean, however, that there are no finer differences between the modes of appearance of after-images at parts of the retina stimulated differently. If we limit ourselves to the last experiments with circular after-images, those after-images which appear nearer than the ground have a somewhat more stable structure than the ground. On the other hand, when the ground lies in front of the after-image, it seems, at least in its central parts, to have greater stability than the after-image lying

---

[1] F. Hillebrand, *Zsch. f. Psychol.*, 1893, 5.

behind it. Even in these cases, however, we can never apprehend the after-image or the ground as a surface colour. These, like other similar observations reported above, simply show that there are different degrees of looseness of a film colour. In spite of the vagueness with which both after-image and ground are localized, there is a certain relationship between the positions of the two *in relation to each other,* i.e., *film colours which are, in themselves, localized indefinitely may be localized fairly definitely with reference to each other.*

The following experiment shows how a familiar form may repress localizing motives rising from attributes of the colour itself. Upon a neutral grey background I pasted a circle consisting of two white and two black quadrants. The negative after-image appeared as a circular area with quadrants which were different in colour, *the entire area, however, lying against a grey background.* The fact that the quadrants belonged to a circle conquered the impression of a difference in distance, which, according to our earlier experiments, the after-images of the different quadrants would tend to arouse. The circle had, as such, higher figural insistence.

Certain spatial arrangements in the presentation, which we should most expect to determine localization in the resulting reproduction, failed to have such an influence. Two observations illustrate this. The observer looked through a round aperture in a white screen at a black area behind it. The after-image was a white circle before a darker background. The fact that the area producing the after-image lay behind the ground has, therefore, obviously no influence at all upon the localization of the after-image. The observers gave the same judgment about the position of a dark after-image upon a bright ground whether it was produced in this way or owed its origin to the exposition of a white circle upon a black background.

In the studies cited above, Rubin refers to the observations reported on the preceding pages. "According to the whole description and to my own experience, I think I am right in assuming that the field which appeared nearer was experienced as figure, the field which appeared farther away as ground. . . . The greater stability of the nearer field, and thus its greater

similarity to surface colour than the more distant field, agrees
with the fact that in the case of surface colours the field which
is apprehended as ground is filmier than the figure." [1]

Projection of Circular After-images upon the Sky.—The
colour of the blue or uniformly clouded sky is not everywhere of the same mode of appearance. Its sponginess
increases, in general, from horizon to zenith. For the
projection of after-images, I selected a region of the sky
midway between horizon and zenith. I made detailed
observations only of after-images produced by fixating
a white circle on a black background or a black circle on
a white background. In spite of the high intrinsic
brightness of the sky, the after-images were sufficiently
distinct. The brighter after-image *always* lies, for all
observers, in front of the rest of the sky; in most cases,
the darker after-image also lies in front of it. These
results correspond, to a certain extent, to what we found
with closed eyes. They indicate that we may ascribe to
the colours of the visual field when the eyes are closed
essentially the same mode of appearance as that of the
sky, *i.e.*, the character of film colour. If the colours seen
when the eyes are closed stood significantly nearer the
surface colours, we should expect other modes of localization in their after-images. Under these conditions, it
seems legitimate to assume that the modes of localization
of after-images projected upon the sky may be explained
in the same way as those appearing when the eyes are
closed. Our assertion that two indefinitely localized film
colours may still have a relatively definite localization *in
reference to each other* is thus confirmed.

The insistence of (surface) colours appears to have an effect
similar to that described in the foregoing experiments upon
the type of localization of colours. Experiments performed
by Fröbes, Jacobsohn and Heine [2] show that of two colours, the
one of *greater insistence* generally tends to stand out before the
other.

[1] E. Rubin, *Visuell wahrgenommene Figuren*, p. 90.
[2] J. Fröbes, *Zsch. f. Psychol.*, 1904, 36; S. Jacobsohn, *Zsch. f. Psychol.*,
1906, 43, 1. Abt., p. 38; R. Heine, *Zsch. f. Psychol.*, 1910, 54, 1. Abt., p. 66.

Advancing and Retreating Colours.—The fact that the chromatic aberration of the human eye is not generally noticeable is presumably due primarily to certain compensatory physiological effects. It appears only under certain particular conditions. The phenomenon of advancing and retreating colours is, as we know, often attributed to it.[1] I believe, however, that the " physical " explanation of advancing and retreating colours must be supplemented from the psychological side. The differing affective value of the chromatic colours, reaching the greatest contrasts in red and blue, has always been recognized and, as we know, is of some significance in Goethe's theory of colour, with his distinction between active and passive colours. The (yellowish) red seems to " bore into the eye." On the other hand, " just as we like to pursue a pleasant object moving away from us, so we like to look at blue, not because it is pressing in upon us, but because it draws us after it." [2] The difference in obtrusiveness between red and blue can escape no observer.[3] This difference in insistence is, it seems to me, the basis for the fact that even if we rule out the topographic factors ordinarily causing them to be seen as nearer, reds seem to stand nearer to us than blues.

I drove a row of broad-headed nails into a dark grey board, so that all the nails stood out equally far from the board. On these nails I pasted alternately red and blue paper squares of high saturation, at distances apart of about 3 mm. When I looked at these papers binocularly from a distance of about 80 cm., the reds stood to a surprising degree (approximately ½–1 cm.) nearer than the blues. The illusion is not so strong monocularly.[4] The strength of the illusion may be changed, under monocular fixation, if we so modify the situation that the colours make an essentially different impression, even though we

---

[1] Helmholtz, II, p. 156 ff. ; E. Brücke, *Sitz.-Ber. der. kaiserl. Akad. d· Wiss. in Wien.*, 1868, 58, Abt. 2, p. 321 ff., and *Die Physiologie der Farben für die Zwecke des Kunstgewerbes.* Leipzig, 1887, p. 173 ff.

[2] *Farbenlehre.* 6. Abt. (" Sinnlich-sittliche Wirkung der Farben ").

[3] Cf., *e.g.*, G. T. Fechner, *Vorschule der Aesthetik.* Leipzig, 1876, 2. Teil, p. 219.

[4] Einthoven, *Arch. f. Ophthalm.*, 1895, 31 ; also in *Brain*, 1893.

do not interfere with the retinal relationships. Thus the red, under monocular fixation and light adaptation, scarcely advances at all if, by means of an episcotister, we reduce considerably the effect of the two colours upon the eye. In this reduction of the light-intensities, the red appears definitely to lose more in insistence than does the blue. If we look at the colours under reduced intensity of illumination and with a dark-adapted eye, so that the Purkinje effect is manifested in a loss of saturation of the red, the blue surfaces seem somewhat nearer than the red. In so far as the retinal relations are concerned, there is certainly no change which might account for a direct reversal of the illusion. The relationship of the colours in insistence has been reversed, and the contours of the coloured surfaces are projected so indistinctly on the eye that they no longer determine localization.

I punched two holes about $\frac{1}{4}$ cm. in diameter and about $\frac{1}{2}$ cm. apart in a piece of white cardboard. The observer, about 60 cm. away, looked through these holes, fixating their borders, at a piece of red or blue paper. The papers were about 50 cm. behind the cardboard and completely filled the apertures; they appeared as film colours. Even in this case the more insistent red seems to lie nearer than the blue. Here, where the edge of the holes is seen distinctly, we cannot, of course, speak of any influence upon localization brought about by different accommodation.

In her study of advancing colours, Belajew-Exemplarsky arrived at the following conclusions : " The advancing character of reds and yellows is almost incontestable, at least in comparison with the other chromatic colours." " In the majority of cases, the chromatic colours seem to lie nearer than the achromatic, if the latter are perceived as such." [1] Matthaei reports that advancing and retreating cease entirely, or at least are strongly reduced, if chromatic colours are presented separately upon equally bright backgrounds.[2]

---

[1] *Zsch. f. Psychol.*, 1925, 96.
[2] R. Matthaei, *Die Welt der Farbe*. Bonn, 1927.

§ 12. The Localization of Film Colours : Rôle of Neighbouring Surfaces

In our distinction of film and surface colours, we have ascribed *in general* to the former an essentially frontal-parallel orientation, while the surface colours may appear in all possible modes of orientation. The question regarding the orientation of film colours requires special study. It appears to be true that a spectral colour fills up the visual field in a frontal-parallel plane. The colour of the sky also seems, for the most part, to have such an orientation. The orientation is not always, however, frontal-parallel, for under some conditions the sky may appear in a different orientation. In what follows we are not limiting ourselves to the orientation of the sky ; this simply serves as an example of film colour. Our experiments are intended to answer this question : How is the localization (distance and orientation) of a film colour influenced by the surface colours in its neighbourhood ?

We tend to think of the space of the world as unbounded. Immediately perceived space ends with the most distant phenomena of colour. In the open air, the sky forms the most distant colour for a large part of the visual field. The sky does not attain this great distance by virtue of its own nature, for " in opposition to everyday experience, the distance of the sky was always found to be astonishingly slight when it was estimated under the exclusion of all aids, especially when the observer was lying on his back and no other objects were seen." [1] We made the following observations of the sky. I punched in the centre of a sheet of light grey cardboard, which filled a large part of the visual field, a hole about 2 cm. in diameter, and held it about 30 cm. in front of an observer in a frontal-parallel plane. The observer had to judge, while fixating the edge of the hole, where the colour film of the sky appeared. It seems to lie behind the opening at a distance not very great and yet difficult to report, and parallel to the cardboard

[1] Metzger, I, p. 17.

itself. The colour of the sky retains its indefinite position
behind the cardboard when we move the latter to a greater
and greater distance and at the same time make the
opening correspondingly greater.

The definitely localized surface colour of the cardboard
thus manifests a tendency to draw the film colour into
its own plane. The following experiment likewise shows
the great extent to which the localization of a film colour
may be influenced. When an observer looks at a film
colour through a cylindrical tube, the colour seems to
lie farther away than when it is seen through the hole
in the cardboard, which is presented at the same visual
angle and at the same distance as the opening of the tube.
We may so arrange the situation that there is approximately the same difference in brightness between the
film colour and, on the one hand, the parts of the tube
surrounding it or, on the other hand, those of the cardboard. The distinct impression of depth which we get
from the tube in monocular vision leads us to displace
the indefinitely localized film colour to a greater distance
than when we are looking through the aperture in the
cardboard. The influence of a tubular device upon the
depth localization of objects seen through it is familiar,
and is used to heighten the effect of depth in panoramas.
We have demonstrated here the effect of this influence
even upon indefinitely localized film colours.

If we hold an aperture screen in a frontal-parallel
position, the film colour lying behind it also appears to
lie in a frontal-parallel plane. This is no longer the case
when we turn the cardboard through a perceptible angle.
The film colour appearing behind the hole then also
tends to turn in the direction in which the cardboard is
turned. There is no perfect correspondence, however,
for the film colour takes on an orientation lying between
that of the cardboard and the frontal-parallel plane. The
indefinite localization of film colours, which we have
hitherto noted only in connection with depth, thus
proves to be characteristic of its orientation, as long as
this is not in the frontal-parallel plane.

Even when film colours are only partially bounded by surface colours and are not entirely surrounded by them, the latter may have a significant influence upon the distance and orientation of the film colours. Let us consider a distant house standing in a position frontal-parallel to the observer ; now if we look at a small section of the sky above the house, the film of the sky seems to lie in frontal-parallel orientation. The impression changes if we consider the position of the sky behind a considerably nearer surface of cardboard held in the same direction. The parts of the sky near the cardboard tend to *bend in toward it*, so that we get the impression of a slightly *arched* film colour. The parts of the sky which lie farther from the surface tend more and more toward an orientation perpendicular to the line of regard. Let us assume that an observer, in an upright position, is looking at a vertical plane, which is so oriented that, if it were lengthened, it would intersect his median plane at an acute angle. The sky behind this plane will no longer appear to lie in a frontal-parallel orientation, but will approach the orientation of the plane itself, without, however, becoming parallel to it. The parts of the sky behind the nearer parts of the plane will seem to lie nearer to the observer than do the other parts. Our observations lead to this conclusion : Every film colour has, in and of itself, a tendency to appear in frontal-parallel orientation. The distance and orientation of the surface colours which neighbour or entirely enclose the film colours act *assimilatively* upon these same two aspects of the film colours. Under otherwise similar conditions, the film colour appears nearer, the nearer the surface colour acting upon it lies to the observer. In general, the more distinctly the surface colour acting upon it deviates from this orientation, the more the film deviates from the frontal-parallel position. In a certain sense, we may also consider as belonging here the experiment with the luminous line described above, for an assimilative effect upon the distance of the surrounding film colour emanates from the luminous line.

Let us attempt an explanation for our observations. When our eyes are closed, the subjective visual grey has that mode of film-colour localization which appears when we eliminate all determinants of spatial perception which might otherwise be effective. All other localizations of film colour with open eyes are *forced upon them* by attendant circumstances. Film colours, it is true, tend when left to themselves to appear as near as possible to the eye, although they *may* be localized at other distances. They are, in a sense, " homeless " colours, adapting themselves to any kind of situation which provides proper spatial supports. In particular, the assimilation of the localization of film colours to that of surface colours, as actually observed in our experiments, seems to be dictated by a principle which we might call that of *convenient visibility*. I can survey two adjacent planes more easily at a single glance when they are at the same distance than when one of them seems to lie nearer toward me. Now if one, a surface colour, must have a certain distance, while the other, a film colour, may be seen at any distance, the latter will be seen as near to the former as opposite tendencies permit. A similar principle holds for the *orientation* of two planes ; the more similar the orientation of the two is, the easier it is to apprehend them with one glance. The film colour moves from the frontal-parallel orientation toward the orientation of the surface colour, simply because it is easier for us to apprehend it in this way.

PART III

SURFACE COLOURS

CHAPTER I

Achromatic Surface Colours in Achromatic Illumination

§ 13. MODIFICATIONS OF SURFACE COLOUR

EVEN though colours of quite different modes of appearance may, through reduction, be transformed into film colours, that does not mean that a film colour is somehow " contained " in a colour-impression of some other mode of appearance. A surface colour is not a modification of a film colour, nor does the latter form a foundation upon which a volume colour might be built up, etc. It is true, of course, that lustre appears only in conjunction with colours of other modes of appearance, and that transparent colours presuppose surface colours to be seen through them. To this extent it may be said that they do not occur *independently* of others, but they are not strictly modifications of these other colour-impressions. We have genuine modifications of colour only in the case of surface colours appearing under the influence of changes in illumination. All the following experiments are devoted particularly to these. Let us begin with *achromatic* surface colours in achromatic illumination. The colour-series which has hitherto been studied with special interest is the one called by Hering the series of achromatic colours.[1] " We may think of all the achromatic colours as so arranged in series that we find at the one

---

[1] Investigations of the black-white series, particularly of the sensation black, often provide ideal examples of the confusion of psychological, physiological and physical points of view. I consider the discovery that black is a positive colour-sensation to be one of the most fruitful in psychological optics.

75

end-point the purest conceivable black, at the other the purest white, and between them in a continuous sequence all possible degrees of darkness or brightness of black, grey-black, black-grey, grey, white-grey, grey-white and white."[1] v. Kries agrees with Hering's view of the unidimensionality of the continuum of achromatic colours. "There is no modification of grey in which the black and white remain in the same ratio and in which both are uniformly stronger or weaker."[2] G. E. Müller has expressed the same view in his discussions of the quantitative unidimensionality of the black-white series of sensations. Indeed, all the authors who have dealt with the black-white series agree that this series has only one dimension. This view is justified if we limit ourselves to the film or surface colours which may be produced in one particular illumination ; for all film or surface colours appearing in one fixed illumination may actually be arranged in *one* series. If, however, we permit the achromatic illumination to vary freely in intensity, we discover a bidimensionality of achromatic surface colours.

§ 14. THE BASIC EXPERIMENT IN COLOUR-CONSTANCY

There are two fundamentally different ways of judging any sense-impression—the absolute and the relative. For example, I can estimate a particular weight absolutely as one kilogram or, by comparing this weight with others, arrive at a judgment concerning its magnitude. A finer analysis shows that no absolute judgment, taken quite strictly, rests solely upon itself, and that no relative judgment is possible without some reference to absolute judgments. We shall disregard such detailed analyses, for in what follows it is sufficient to take the opposition "absolute-relative" in its grosser but generally understood sense.

---

[1] Hering, VI, p. 25.
[2] J. v. Kries, " Die Gesichtsempfindungen," in W. Nagel's *Handbuch d. Physiol. d. Menschen,* 3. Braunschweig, 1905, p. 142.

In the first experiment to be described we used a chart consisting of forty-eight different achromatic colour-squares, such as those used by Burzlaff.[1] Each colour-square was 6 × 6 cm. in size. The brightest was a good white, the darkest a velvet-black, the other members ranging between these extremes, and all being about equally distant from each other in brightness. The differences in brightness were all supraliminal. The colour-squares were arranged, in order of decreasing whiteness, in twelve rows of four members each upon a neutral grey background 6 × 8 cm. in size. This chart, with its forty-eight steps of grey, is presented in an illumination such as we have in summer about noon under a lightly clouded sky. We may then observe each grey of our scale by itself and characterize it in some way, *e.g.*, by means of language. Let us now think of the observation as repeated at an hour in the afternoon of the same day when the intensity of illumination has sunk to about one-fifth that of the earlier hour. A change of illumination intensity of such magnitude, although it is considerable from the physical point of view, is so slight as regards experience that it may completely escape the naïve consciousness. Now, how are the forty-eight achromatic colours judged in the new illumination ? Is the process more difficult and do the colours appear to be different ? Neither is the case. Judgment is just as easy as before, and the colours do not appear to be changed. We still tend to call the brightest white " white " and the velvet-black " black," and all members lying between them may be well distinguished from each other. Thus it seems as if the character of the colours remained entirely intact under this strong change of illumination. There seems to be an independence of the colours of objects from the change of illumination. Under these conditions, " colour-constancy " appears to be ideal, in the sense that the members of the colour-chart remain identical with themselves with change in the intensity of illumination ; it is as if the difference in

[1] *Zsch. f. Psychol.*, 1931, 109.

illumination were simply suspended. The "invariance" of the colours under change of illumination seems to be total. Should we be content with such conclusions reached through absolute judgments? Obviously not. However valuable this fundamental experiment with absolute judgment of colours may be to demonstrate the problem of colour constancy or colour invariance, the facts must be ascertained in another way—and this other way can be only that of comparison. We must compare with each other visual fields containing colours standing in objectively different illuminations. Only if we find no influence of illumination even in this comparative setting shall we confess that the eye is prepared to suspend an objective difference in illumination. Only if we discover through comparison that achromatic colours are identical in visual fields of different intensities of illumination may we speak of a total colour-constancy. The comparative procedure must be used to supplement absolute judgment not only to decide these open questions but also for other cogent reasons. It is only through confronting visual fields of different illuminations that we may realize the influences of adaptive adjustments of the eye upon the experimental results and determine the various contrast relationships which may be effective. Only the comparative procedure makes it possible to determine the limits of apparently total colour-constancy under variations of intensity of illumination, limits which we assumed to be 1 : 5 in the basic experiment. In short, only a comparative procedure permits exact measurements. The dependence of the experimental results upon the experimental method in this field had not, until recently, been investigated, and yet it is a question of the greatest significance. Burzlaff has made a thorough-going study of this question; we shall report the results in detail in § 30. There it will be shown how questions of method run in striking parallelism to questions of organization of the field.

In one of Jaensch's articles we find the following statements: "If only one kind of illumination is present at one time, it is almost completely taken into account, and therefore colour-constancy is approximately total. . . . The most important cases of transformation provided in everyday life are of this type, *e.g.*, when we move from near the window to the farther side of a room or when the total illumination changes."[1] Marzynski speaks of a total transformation when the intensity of illumination changes in the entire room ; otherwise he speaks of a partial transformation.[2]

§ 15. ILLUMINATION PERSPECTIVE IN ARTIFICIAL LIGHT

A strong light was set up about two metres above the floor on the wall of a dark-room. The observer sat under the lamp in such a position that we might present coloured papers to him at distances up to about five metres. We used a series of eighteen achromatic papers differing from each other in brightness by about the same amounts ; the terminals of the series were a velvet-black and a very bright white. We held this series one metre away from the observer, perpendicular to the light-rays. Then we set up individually papers of the same brightness as those of the series at a distance of about 5 metres from the observer, and had him compare these with the papers of the series. If the paper in the back of the room were of greatest whiteness, and the observer had to locate this in the series one metre from him, he decided in most cases upon a position between the second and third members. We now had the observer select from a series of achromatic papers one which was, qualitatively, like the paper in the back of the room. Now there were two papers at different distances from the light-source which were judged equally white, although the nearer reflected about twenty times as much light as the more distant. It is true that the two papers did not appear alike in every respect ; the nearer presented

[1] E. R. Jaensch, *Sitzungsberichte d. Ges. zur Beförderung d. ges. Naturw. zu Marburg*, 1917, p. 5.
[2] *Zsch. f. Psychol.*, 1921, 87.

a white of greater " pronouncedness." We might be tempted to speak of a difference in the intensity of the whites. I prefer, however, for certain reasons, to be content with the expression " degrees of pronouncedness of the same white."[1] It is also easy to demonstrate degrees of pronouncedness lying between these two whites. If we gradually move the white surface from the farther position to the nearer, we see approximately the same white, but its pronouncedness is gradually increasing. (There is also a change in quality, the surface becoming somewhat whiter when it is nearer. We shall disregard here this qualitative change.)

We might be inclined, in the experiment reported, to call both papers equally white, but the nearer " brighter," and the more distant " darker." If we were to accept this terminology corresponding to ordinary usage, we should have to speak of qualitatively the same white assuming different brightnesses. The only objection to such terminology is really that the concept of " brightness " is already used in another sense in the psychology of colour, for ordinarily we speak of a chromatic colour as being brighter or darker according to the particular member of the black-white series with which it is correlated. We shall return later to the question of the brightness of a colour in connection with other experiments of the same kind (§ 36).

---

[1] " Bühler believed that pronouncedness was the long-sought intensity of colours. Katz, however, rejects Bühler's concept of intensity . . . since, according to other statements of Bühler, a strongly illuminated black should be called more intense, while a black in reduced illumination is more pronounced. . . . We should not try to apply to Katz's findings those categories which we used to apply in discussing the old problem of attributes in the theory of sensations, i.e., in discussing the question of the immanent and essential attributes of a sensation (Stumpf). The various conceptual attempts at systematization connected with these matters presuppose an abstract concept of sensation which has, through the important findings of Katz, become problematic " (Gelb, p. 617). Müller says, in connection with my findings about the degrees of pronouncedness in the black-white series : " In this discussion, the author recognizes the correctness of our own view that in establishing those various degrees of pronouncedness of a black-white sensation we are dealing with ' the perception of different degrees of intensity of the same quality ' " (Müller, III). " There are still other . . . cases in which . . . the various nuances of grey and white permit us to apprehend a variability in their insistence and intensity." " In his haploscopic experiments on convergence-micropsia, Jaensch (1911) came to the conclusion that when the angle of convergence of the ocular axes increases, the insistence of a colour increases, its hue, brightness and saturation remaining unchanged " (Müller, III).

The question arises whether, in our experiment, some physiological factors may not transform the ratio of 1 : 20 in physical intensities of light into a different ratio. We are referring to the possible influence of the width of the pupil as well as of adaptive readjustments of the retina. In answer, we might mention the following : (a) We may perform the experiment even with pupils which have artificially been kept small ; the result is not changed. Kravkov has repeated experiments with an atropinized eye. It appears that " the pupillary reflex plays no rôle in the occurrence of transformation phenomena." [1] (b) Since adaptation depends only upon the *peripheral* intensity of excitation, and the same thing holds for the pupillo-motor valence of a light, the physiological effect of our two papers is really determined only by their physical light-intensities. Thus physiological relationships do not act in the direction of a qualitative constancy.

The next question concerns the appearance of different degrees of pronouncedness in other members of the black-white series. The hypothesis that a similar state of affairs holds for colours standing near white as for white itself is confirmed when we repeat with light greys the experiments already carried out with white ; we discover then, however, that the greys do not show different degrees of pronouncedness as clearly as does the white. If we pass to darker members of the series, we reach a region where it is doubtful whether the nearer or the more distant member represents the particular grey quality in greater pronouncedness. As for the most extreme black and the colours near it, there seems to be no question that they may appear in distinctly different degrees of pronouncedness under the given experimental conditions. But now, in contrast to the experiments with white, the *more distant* papers show the colour qualities in higher degrees of pronouncedness. In all cases, however, the nearer of two such colours has the greater insistence. In the case of the colours belonging to the white end of the scale, higher pronouncedness coincides with higher insistence ; for black and its neighbouring colours this relationship does not hold. We

[1] *Arch. f. d. ges. Psychol.*, 48, 1924.

F

must therefore guard against a confusion between "insistence" and "pronouncedness."

According to the observations described above, it is certain that achromatic surface colours appear in various degrees of pronouncedness. The bi-dimensionality of the continuum of achromatic surface colours is thus also demonstrated; for, according to these considerations, we are free to pass from a given member of the black-white series to colours qualitatively different or to colours showing the same quality in different pronouncedness. This result is to be considered a consequence of the comparison of colours belonging to differently illuminated visual fields. Absolute judgment of colours in a single visual field with unitary illumination causes us too easily to overlook the fact that the degree of pronouncedness with which colours appear under such conditions is only one among many possibilities. We see that it would be false to conclude from a fundamental experiment such as the one described above that there is an ideal colour constancy.

Probably the unjustified identification of the two cases (1) in which white passes through steps of grey with constant intensity of illumination, and (2) in which it passes into "lightlessness" with approximately the same quality under reduction of the intensity of illumination of the visual field, is not without significance for an understanding of the disputed question whether black is the least quantity of white or whether it is a unique quality.

§ 16. Genuine Colour and Normal Illumination

In dealing with spatial perspective, we distinguish the concepts of *real* size (or form) of objects, their *apparent* size (or form) and their size (or form) *upon the retina*. It is possible to form three analogous concepts for a certain sphere of colour-experiences. 1. It is customary to speak of the genuine or real colour of an object. I shall try later to make this concept more precise. 2. There are certain objections against speaking of "physiological colour," and yet there is some value in correlating a particular retinal process with each colour experience. Unfortunately, it is not as simple to characterize this process as to determine the retinal image corresponding to an external object ; the various procedures of reduction, however, give us some information concerning whether the retinal processes corresponding to various impressions are alike or not. 3. We have still to introduce the concept of apparent colour. If I move an achromatic surface to different distances from a light-source, I know very well that the colour-impression which I observe is only *apparent*; I know that under these conditions the " genuine " or " real " colour of the surface does not change, white remaining white and black remaining black. We shall call the immediately perceived (not the inferred) colour of the paper as seen at any time in any illumination, together with its quality and pronouncedness, its " apparent " colour. Just as apparent size points beyond itself to real size and apparent form to real form, an apparent colour has intentional character ; its reference is to genuine colour.

We believe that we apprehend the *genuine* colour of an object only under certain particular conditions of illumination. Neither twilight nor direct sunlight presents the genuine colour of an object. We must rather choose an intensity of illumination such as there is in the open air when the sky is lightly clouded. We shall call such intensity of illumination *normal* illumination. It is not characterized by a single value but by a certain range of values. In what follows, whenever we speak for the sake of simplicity of *normal* illumination, we shall mean this range. Is the uniqueness of this illumination apprehended through certain attributes of the colour-matter of the impression ? Detailed study leads us to a negative answer. Colours in normal illumination do not differ in any unique sense from colours appearing under other intensities of illumination. The only attributes in which a colour impression may stand out absolutely from others is that of a particularly high or low insistence. The illumination intensity in which colours have a high insistence is *not* that of normal but of a higher illumination, while the subjective grey has the *lowest* insistence of all colours. Perhaps it is not superfluous to remark that in general we can never ascribe to a colour an attribute of distinctness. In the case of a saturated red containing a little blue, I may speak of *distinctness* in reference to its red component, of *indistinctness* in reference to its blue or achromatic component. If, however, we exclude comparison with series of colours and thereby exclude all questions of redness, whiteness, etc., there is no meaning in speaking generally of a distinct or indistinct colour. This consideration should lead us to discard the view that the colours of objects have, in normal illumination, a special degree of distinctness.

"Normal" illumination is not rooted in the colour-values as such, but owes its unique position to other factors. Even surfaces which have the greatest uniformity of colouring show minute differences in colour which become bearers of surface structure or, to use a good term introduced by Bühler, of microstructure. If we are able to judge correctly the objects around us, it is of great importance that we apprehend the material of which they consist. Since the eye cannot penetrate into opaque objects, it must be limited to characteristics of their superficial structure, in so far as it can get any information at all about the material of the objects. This superficial structure is revealed most distinctly under certain particular conditions of illumination; hence if we wish to know the material of an object, we carry it into an illumination which is optimal for the apprehension of its surface structure. Only the colours of objects which appear under such conditions of illumination should be *distinguished especially* from other colour-experiences. They function as the *genuine* colours of objects and become representative of them. Accordingly, we need only to answer the question as to which illuminating conditions are most favourable for the perception of microstructures. We learn from Hering's studies that there is an optimal illumination for the cognition of forms. " The distinctness of vision reaches its *absolute maximum*, after adaptation, only in a certain degree of illumination, which we may call the *absolute optimal illumination*. Everyone knows from his own experience that there is for the eye a degree of illumination in which he sees most distinctly, distinguishes objects with least difficulty and perceives most details in them, and that any illumination falling considerably below or rising considerably above this optimum reduces markedly the distinctness of vision." [1] For most individuals with normal eyesight, this absolute optimal illumination would seem to lie at that illumination characterized as normal. If the normal intensity of illumination gives way to a higher or lower illumination, the genuine colours of objects are no longer seen, since the details of microstructure have receded. The perceptibility of a microstructure in its details leads us to accept the illumination as normal, even if other factors otherwise affording knowledge of the illuminating conditions are lacking or are artificially excluded.[2] Under natural conditions of living, a fading of microstructure will appear much more frequently and in a more striking degree as a result of a decrease than as a result of an increase in intensity of illumination. When factors ordinarily determining the impression of intensity of illumination are excluded, the perception of indefiniteness of microstructure is in most cases bound up with an experience of reduced intensity of illumination. The only really unambiguous relationship between intensity of illumination and degree of distinctness of microstructure is that between normal illumination and maximal distinctness. We shall learn later [3] of a particular factor which is important in the apprehension of the absolute intensity of illumination in a visual field. Although the degree of distinctness of

[1] Hering, VI, p. 73.
[2] *Cf.* the observations in § 43 in which peripheral vision is excluded.
[3] *Cf.* § 65.

microstructure provides no clear-cut measure for this, it does furnish a motive for apprehending as the *same* the illumination within the entire visual field or a region of it, in so far as the microstructures of the objects within it are equally distinct or vague. We shall discover this motive in many cases. It is perhaps not superfluous to add that in the indissoluble intertwining of illumination and object colour, normal illumination and genuine colour also form an indissoluble experiential unity.

Kaila has raised an objection against my view that normal illumination is a phenomenal datum. " Katz speaks of normal illumination as a phenomenal datum in the same sense as of abnormal illuminations. . . . I should like, on the contrary, to defend the thesis that normal illumination is not a phenomenal datum in the same sense as are abnormal illuminations. . . . Optimal illumination is characterized by the fact that surface colours appear pure and unveiled, undisturbed by shadows, clouds, lustrous lights or reflections." [1] It is quite correct to say that in normal illumination surface colours are seen as pure and unveiled ; it is, indeed, for this reason that I speak of the genuine colour which is revealed in normal illumination. We must, however, contradict the statement that normal illumination is not a phenomenal datum. It is the illumination of greatest definiteness, and in no other does the radiating light of empty space appear so clearly. If Kaila were right, the experience of illumination would have higher phenomenal reality the more it deviated from the normal illumination, and thus we should have to consider an illumination such as prevails in an unilluminated dark-room as the prototype of the experience of illumination.

Surface structure or microstructure must be distinguished from " material " structure, *i.e.*, from that special formation of microstructure which informs us about the material of which an object consists. We see whether an object is made of wood, stone, cloth, etc., and after some practice we even recognize the particular kind of wood,

[1] *Psychol. Forsch.*, 1923, 3.

stone, cloth, etc. What leads to this recognition of various materials is, to a certain extent, grounded in that impression of the microstructure which, in the case of all substances, gives an indication of materiality as such. If we expose on the same background minute particles of various materials (wood, paper, stone, coal), we recognize material particles, but not the material of which they consist.

I have developed the theory of material structure further in my book on touch, and I consider my findings so important in the present context that it seems appropriate to give some of them here. We encounter all materials in natural or in artificial forms. A rock which has developed naturally has natural form, a plate polished by the human hand artificial form. We must confess that it is not always easy to decide whether we are dealing with a natural or an artificial form, but as a rule it is possible to make the distinction, a distinction which is not unimportant for our orientation in the external world. If a wooden board is lying before me, I apprehend its material immediately in normal illumination. This apprehension is quite independent of the artificial colour given to the wood, provided that there is no superimposed colour which completely hides the grain. The board might shine in all the colours of the rainbow, and yet the structure " wood " would be everywhere evident. The recognition of material is also independent of the external formation of the wood; it makes no difference whether the board has large flat surfaces or curved surfaces, or whether the carpenter has given it an elaborate form. The material structure is shown at every point of the artificial form. How, now, is this material structure presented ? Description faces serious difficulties, and I must here beg the reader to co-operate with me by observing carefully the material structure of the printed page before him. There is a certain distance of the eye from the paper at which the structure appears most clearly ; we can determine it without much difficulty. We then discover formal elements, very small and hardly demarcated from each other, which owe their visibility to minimal differences in brightness and hue. These elements are so small that we might very well discover multitudes of them within a square millimetre. There is an astonishing variety among these elements ; even with rather careful inspec-

tion we do not find two (marked off from each other with
some arbitrariness) which are completely alike, and yet there
is, in spite of all this irregularity, a certain regularity in the
recurrence of the elements over the entire surface. There is,
so to say, a type of element which is bearer of the impression
" paper of this sort." We might even say that regularity within
irregularity of elements is the law of material structure. There
are materials in which the smallest formal elements are combined
into structures of higher order, and these in turn into structures
of still higher order; we may think of the transition from the
smallest elements in wood to suggested grain and then to the
distinct grain shown by the annual rings. Depending upon
the circumstances in which the judgment is to be made, we
find support, in our orientation concerning material, in the
elements or in the higher structures of one order or another.
The structural elements may determine our judgment about
material even if we are not really conscious of them. The
differences in colour and brightness which make up the
structural elements of the paper have no weight in the judgment
of the colour of the paper. Following Hering, we may say
that a coloured paper mounted on glass has ideal uniformity
of colour; yet even in this case, those differences of colour and
brightness are not entirely lacking, for otherwise it would be
seen no longer as paper but only as a coloured " something "
occupying space.

If a certain artificial form is impressed upon a material, new
structures of formal elements, different from those of the
natural form, come into being. These structures may themselves be extraordinarily small; we may think, *e.g.*, of the very
fragile materials woven from silk. Yet they are always larger
than the elements which are characteristic of the material
itself (*e.g.*, silk). The elements of natural and artificial form
differ, however, not only in size but also in the respect that the
elements of artificial forms show a much greater regularity.

Against our view that the normal illumination of an
object is determined by the maximal degree of distinctness of its microstructure, it is unjustified to bring the
objection that this degree of distinctness depends upon
the distance between the eye and the coloured object,
and that therefore the judgment as to whether or not
an illumination is normal is subject to differences in

distance; for we mean, obviously, the maximum of distinctness under otherwise equal conditions, *i.e.*, with the same distances of the surfaces from the eye. The relationship between the degree of distinctness of microstructure and the distance from which it is perceived follows a rigid law, and there is even evidence that it is a " law of structure " in v. Kries's sense.

When, with increasing distance, microstructure loses distinctness or even disappears entirely, there appear in its place other characteristics giving us the consciousness of materiality—finer or grosser contours, which may appear in various degrees of distinctness, depending upon distance. Finally, perhaps only a vague outline of an object may guarantee its apprehension as a material thing. Let us now consider an object presented in normal illumination with varying claims to distinctness of surface structure or other attributes essential for its materiality, depending upon the distance at which the object is presented. The distinctness with which the microstructure of an object is seen may thus become zero without our losing the impression that we are seeing an object colour. A distant house-wall does not need to show any more surface structure than does the blue sky ; yet, on account of its perception as a thing with certain properties—a perception guaranteed by its framing contours and its meaningful setting in the whole visual perceptual complex—its colour will be more related to object colour than to the optical *quale* of the sky. I must, of course, add that the impression of *distinct* object colour is bound up with the perception of microstructure. Hence, in any case in which the distinctness of structure is reduced, either by an increase in the distance of the coloured surface or by a peculiarity of illumination, the impression comes more or less to resemble that of a filmy or " free " colour.

1. Let us consider an object, such as a black hat, which has a dark colour in normal illumination. If we reduce the intensity of illumination, the black which we then perceive may be of greater pronouncedness than the black seen in normal illumina-

tion. We ascribe to the hat as its genuine colour, however, not this black of higher pronouncedness but the black of lower pronouncedness seen in normal illumination. A white paper does not reveal its genuine colour in sunlight, although under such circumstances the white may be much more pronounced than in normal illumination. The genuine colour of an object is thus not always perceived in that intensity of illumination in which it possesses a relatively high degree of pronouncedness.

2. We may mention here one of Gelb's experiments, which shows the great significance of microstructure for the judgment both of object colour and of the illumination presented with it. The strong light of an arc-lamp is thrown upon a velvet-black disc in a weakly illuminated dark-room. Even if we look at the disc from a very short distance, it appears white as long as it is rotating. If we stop the movement of the disc, its colour is suddenly transformed into black and at the same time we see it as strongly illuminated, while during the rotation it appeared weakly illuminated. "As soon as the disc stands still, the small particles of dust and the fibres of the velvet-black which reflect more light than the background become visible, and the visibility of these lighter particles (microstructure) brings about the alteration described." [1]

The intensity of illumination which we have called " normal " might, of course, be simply the most common illumination. We might think of defining as " normal " that intensity of illumination which prevails most of the time when we are perceiving objects, and as the "genuine" colours of objects those which we have perceived most frequently. It is to be granted that the prevalence of normal illumination is not without significance. Yet it is difficult to explain many facts [2] unless we assume that normal illumination is anchored in the degree of distinctness of surface structure. The preponderance of normal illumination in time is not a sufficient explanation for its unique status. It is conceivable, on the other hand, that the temporal preponderance of (essentially) achromatic daylight over chromatic types of illumination appearing in life contributes to the fact that we ascribe to objects as their genuine colours those which they manifest in

---

[1] Gelb, p. 675.   [2] Cf., e.g., Chapter II.

a certain *achromatic* daylight illumination. The qualitative changes which daylight undergoes in the course of a day are of slight significance compared with the considerable changes in its intensity. Natural chromatic illuminations of high intensity are extremely rare, while most of our artificial light-sources have marked chromatic valences.

If I illuminate the same paper partly with daylight and partly with chromatic artificial light, so that its variously illuminated parts look equally bright, I believe that in general, with a light-adapted eye, I see more distinctly the microstructure of the part struck by daylight. To make this observation it is convenient to use a paper-covered wedge (Bouguer's photometer), one side of which is turned toward an artificial source of chromatic illumination, the other subjected to direct daylight. According to the criterion which we established above for normal illumination (the illumination most favourable for perception of microstructure), daylight may be called normal in comparison with other kinds of illumination.

I shall not pursue here the interconnection between distinctness of microstructure and visual acuity as illumination is varied. Most of the experiments concerning these relationships which are free from objections on the side of method have been carried out with approximately monochromatic illumination. There is, however, no complete unanimity in the results. While, for example, A. Boltunow[1] found the least acuity for red, a moderate acuity for green, and the highest acuity for white, L. Löser[2] found, on the contrary, that acuity in green illumination was superior to that in white.

§ 17. Surface Colour and the Recognition of Objects

We have sensations not for the sake of themselves but for the sake of the services which they perform for us in our orientation in the external world. " Seeing is not

[1] *Zsch. f. Sinnesphysiol.*, 1908, 42.   [2] *Arch. f. Ophth.*, 1909, 69.

a matter of looking at light-waves as such, but of looking at external things mediated by these waves; the eye has to instruct us, not about the intensity or quality of the light coming from external objects at any one time, but about these objects themselves." [1] We agree with this view; yet it is true that we cannot ascribe recognition value to all the colour-experiences lying within the great manifold of colours. We may contrast film and surface colours in this respect. [2] Surface colours represent qualities of objects taken to be invariable. In unbiassed observation of objects, we also experience at every moment the type and intensity of the dominant illumination. Illumination causes innumerable modifications of surface colours to appear. A film colour, on the other hand, is subject to no such modifications; it does not point, in the same sense as does a surface colour, to an objective bearer, and accordingly does not represent any fixed quality of colour. When I perceive a film colour by looking at a coloured object through a reduction screen, and then throw a shadow or a light upon the object, the film appearing in the aperture will, of course, appear darker or lighter, but there is no meaning in speaking of a shadowed or lighted film colour. The *neighbourhood* of the film colour may appear in a particular illumination, but this illumination does not extend to the film colour itself, as long as it is really apprehended as a film colour. If we radiate the closed eyelid with light, we may judge conclusively that our eyelid is illuminated, and can even denote as " luminous " the colour experienced in this situation; but we cannot say that the film colour which we perceive under these conditions has assumed a particular *illumination*. The severance of illumination and illuminated object vanishes in the case of an individual film colour. Film colours are without very great significance for orientation with reference to the colour-relationships of the external world.

[1] Hering, VI, p. 23.
[2] Lustre frequently gives important information about the material and surface character of objects. *Cf.* W. Schapp, *Beiträge zur Phäno-menologie der Wahrnehmung*, Göttingen Dissertation, 1910, pp. 76–98.

They tend to be taken, as they appear, "as space-filling *quale*"; they are, to a certain extent, stopgaps. So many factors determine the particular colour which appears in the reduction screen that it is quite impossible, from an observation of the colour alone, to determine its real locus in space.

If we reduce the same light by achromatic screens of the same quality but of different pronouncedness, can we perceive the same achromatic film colour in different degrees of pronouncedness? I have found, as a rule, that whenever this question has been answered in the affirmative, the reduced colour has not been perceived as a film but rather as a surface. Particularly when the illumination is strongly increased or diminished, and the surface structure of the reduction screen thereby becomes less distinct, there is a tendency for reduction screen and reduced colour to assume the same mode of appearance, *i.e.*, the film colour tends to look more surfacy. Also we have already learned, as a matter of fact, that a film colour may assume the character of surface colour as a result of a change in attitude. At the moment of that change, the colour ceases to follow laws of film and obeys, rather, those of surface.[1]

Although, in accordance with general linguistic usage, we speak of sensations of colour, we realize quite clearly that this usage is not entirely unobjectionable. "To call colours 'sensations' is not in accord with the original meaning of the word 'sensation.' In the strict sense of the word, a 'sensation' is something which we experience in or on the surface of the body. Colours, however, always appear outside of our bodies and, in particular, outside of our eyes." [2] I may refer here to a discussion in my book on touch concerning the objective character of colour-impressions in contrast to the bipolarity of touch impressions.

---

[1] We may refer here to Cassirer's important discussion of the epistemological significance of the film-surface distinction. E. Cassirer, *Philosophie der symbolischen Formen*. III. Teil: *Phänomenologie der Erkenntnis*. Berlin, 1929, p. 151 ff.

[2] Hering, VI, p. 4.

§ 18. The Reduction of Colours to the Same Illumination

In reduction to the same mode of appearance (§ 9) we have an instrument for unifying the modes of appearance of colour-impressions. At the same time, we may consider this reduction as a means of *unifying conditions of illumination*. Looking through the reduction screen causes the film colours seen to appear in a visual field of the same illumination—that of the reduction screen; in referring to this effect, we shall speak of a *reduction to the same illumination*. It is true that two surface colours no longer appear to be illuminated at all after complete reduction, yet they no longer appear *differently* illuminated. We should not overlook the fact that in reduction we perceive at least the reduction screen in a certain illumination. *Thus we are able, by means of a reduction screen, to mask a particular illumination; but as long as any surface colour at all is present in the visual field, we can never eliminate illumination altogether.* It would, therefore, be false to say that reduction gives us, to a certain extent, the retinal excitation itself; it is, rather, quite certain that, even under reduction, the illumination perceived in the visual field is a factor in determining the colour-impression.[1] In the present experiments, the unification of illumination reached through reduction is a unification in terms of normal illumination. We should remark here, however, that unification of illumination is possible in other directions; we shall use this technique in later experiments.

Fuchs has this to say of reduction from the point of view of the *gestalt* theory : " From the point of view of the *gestalt* theory, the reductive type of perception consists in the production of certain particular configural impressions, the preceding configurations having been destroyed. Hence the colours also assume a different

---

[1] " We must emphasize the fact that when we use a hole in a screen, there is no retinal vision in the sense of pure sensation ; Katz has already pointed this out." Gelb, p. 669.

appearance."[1] We shall devote a particular section to the relationships between the *gestalt* theory and the phenomena of colour constancy.

§ 19. ILLUMINATION PERSPECTIVE IN DAYLIGHT

In a room lighted by a window there prevails a distribution of light similar to that which was provided in the artificially lighted dark-room for the experiments of § 15. In such a room the intensity of illumination decreases as the distance from the window increases. In the open air, the colour of a piece of paper appears about equally bright and equally pronounced when it is seen from different distances, because there the distribution of light is essentially uniform. What we call illumination perspective holds for daylight only in the case of a room illuminated from one side. The following experiments were performed in a room with two windows, one of which was covered completely, the other partly covered by a roller-blind.

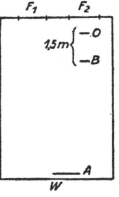

FIG. I

The observer sat near the window F_2, which was only partially covered by the blind (Fig. 1). A colour-wheel B stood in approximately normal illumination about 1·5 m. from the window. Any colours with any backgrounds might be set up upon it. Close by the wall W of the room there was a second wheel A. The colour upon it had for its background a bright grey surface covering the wall W. The distance between A and the window was about 5 m. In all the experiments the background of the disc B was equated in light-intensity to disc A. Disc B, which served as a comparison disc, had a diameter of about 10 cm. The diameter of disc A was chosen so large that it appeared under approximately the

[1] Fuchs, I, p. 190.

same visual angle as *B*. This was done to equate the contrast relationships for the two discs. For some observers, the achromatic papers on disc *A* (standard disc) had a tinge of orange. When this was the case, the same hue was produced upon disc *B* by the addition of orange. The white valences of these chromatic colours were taken into account.

The following set of instructions was given: " A certain achromatic colour is presented on disc *A*. Your problem is to find a colour of the same quality upon disc *B*. *Make your judgment only on the basis of your immediate impression, not on the basis of any reflection about the type of illumination of the discs.*" We must emphasize here and in similar later experiments that we do not mean by establishment of equations between two colour-impressions those identities which are usual in most experiments in the physiology of colour. Here we have an equation between two colours only in one particular respect, while in other respects an inequality remains. The method of limits, with both increasing and decreasing series, was used. The principal values represent arithmetic means of three upper and three lower limiting values. Since the number of experiments was small, I have not given the distributions. They are somewhat large and are of about the same range as the distributions which I shall give later in connection with similar experiments (§ 25). In all the experiments, with the exception of the last, the brightness of disc *B* was changed, a fixed brightness being retained on *A*. In the last experiments, disc *B* contained 360° of black or approximately 358° of black and 2° of red and yellow, and disc *A* was varied.

As we have already said, we may consider the prevailing illumination of *B* as approximately normal. The loss undergone by the light on its way from disc *B* to disc *A* was such that under reduction 360° of white upon *A* appeared equal to 17° of white, 4° of orange and 339° of black upon *B*. If we take into consideration the white-valence of the coloured sector, as well as that of the velvet black, the intensity of the illumination upon disc *A* was about 1/14 that upon disc *B*. The setting which I made was accepted by all the observers. The chromatic component shows that, under these conditions of illumination, the distant white paper had an orange tinge. On each day of the experiment I set up beforehand on disc B the above-mentioned values. If this setting did not appear equal to that of 360° of white upon disc A (the two, of course, being seen after reduction), the height of the blind was changed until equality was noted. This equation guaranteed an approximately constant ratio of illumination intensities of the two discs on the various days of the experiment. To save space, I shall give the numerical values of only one of the four observers.

OBSERVER K

1.	Disc A:	360° W	Disc B:	161·2° W	10·8° R	10·0° Y [1]
2.	,,	270° W	,,	110·0° W	28·7° R	9·0° Y
3.	,,	210° W	,,	92·7° W	5·3° R	8·3° Y
4.	,,	180° W	,,	97·7° W	4·0° R	4·2° Y
5.	,,	155° W	,,	48·5° W	3·7° R	5·0° Y
6.	,,	125° W	,,	38·7° W	3·3° R	2·0° Y
7.	,,	100° W	,,	32·1° W	2·8° R	2·0° Y
8.	,,	80° W	,,	19·7° W	2·8° R	1·7° Y
9.	,,	60° W	,,	11·2° W	3·0° R	1·7° Y
10.	,,	45° W	,,	5·5° W	2·0° R	1·8° Y
11.	,,	22° W	,,	0·0° W	1·0° R	0·5° Y

In the discussion of these results, it will be advantageous to form the quotients of the brightnesses set up on the two discs which appeared qualitatively equal. Here the stimulus-value of 60° of velvet black is set equal to 1° of white. Also we took into account the white-valences of the coloured papers, as determined by means of Hess's method of peripheral values.[2]

1. 174·6 : 360·0 =0·49	6. 48·6 : 128·9 =0·38
2. 132·4 : 271·5 =0·49	7. 39·9 : 104·3 =0·38
3. 103·7 : 212·5 =0·49	8. 27·6 : 84·7 =0·33
4. 88·3 : 183·0 =0·48	9. 19·3 : 65·0 =0·30
5. 57·9 : 158·4 =0·36	10. 13·2 : 50·3 =0·26
	11. 6·5 : 27·6 =0·24

---

[1] W=white; R=red; Y=yellow.
[2] C. Hess, *Arch. f. Ophthalm.*, 1889, 35.

G

We shall call the brightness quotients so obtained the
B-series.

I have emphasized above the general acceptance by all
the observers of the colour equation which I had established under reduction. That implies that the observers
would have accepted each other's equations under
reduction. *Without* reduction, the differences between
the settings made by the four observers are much
greater. To take the extreme cases, for $A = 360° W$,
observer N set up $315° W$ and observer M $127° W$ on
disc B. We shall return to these individual differences
in § 27.

We shall speak of *ideal* colour-constancy when the
judgment correctly indicates the objective relationship
existing between the colours of the papers. If colour-
constancy were ideal in our experiments, *e.g.*, if white
should undergo no qualitative change in addition to its
change in pronouncedness, we should expect the B-
quotients to have the value 1. Instead of this, our
observers gave for $A = 360° W$ the values 0·49, 0·62,
0·36 and 0·88—values representing, in part, quite considerable qualitative changes of the white. Under
the given experimental conditions, the B-quotients fall
below 1 not only for white but for all other achromatic
colours.

Fig. 2 gives graphically the results for observers L and
K. As abscissae we chose the sizes (in degrees) of the
white sectors on A, and as ordinates the B-quotients
corresponding to the various settings. The two curves
take a similar course. At first they remain at about the
same height, and then fall. The meaning is this : *When
the intensity of the illumination is steadily decreased, the
colours which retain their qualitative character most stably
are white and the colours near it ; the influence upon the
qualities of the colours becomes stronger the farther we pass
from white and its neighbouring colours.*[1] We may remark

---

[1] E. R. Jaensch and E. A. Müller have essentially confirmed this finding.
" Apparent change in brightness increases in proportion to the brightness
of the disc." *Zsch. f. Psychol.*, 1920, 83, p. 293.

here, in anticipation, that a similar result was found in other experiments on the influencing of achromatic colours by conditions of illumination. To say that there is a tendency for the curves to drop is not, however, to tell the whole story. This drop is saltatory rather than continuous. We have already referred to the fact that at their beginnings the curves are approximately horizontal—in the case of K up to 180°, in the case of L up to 210°. Now it seems to me that a saltatory rather than continuous decline is to be observed in the further course of the curves. In the case of K, we may make out two

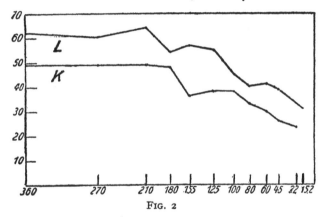

FIG. 2

pronounced groups of values for which the curve is approximately parallel to the X-axis—(1) from 360° to 180°, and (2) from 155° to 100°. We may distinguish three such groups for L—(1) from 360° to 210°; (2) from 180° to 125°; and (3) from 80° to 45°. How can we interpret these groupings? If we run through an achromatic series, we cannot at any point notice anything like a sudden transition. We find, however, a certain articulation within the series when we undertake to combine into groups those members which fall under the rubrics of white, light grey, middle grey, dark grey and black.[1] These are linguistic expressions which are usually

[1] Cf. A. Lehmann, "Über Wiedererkennen," Wundts Philos. Stud., 1889, 5, p. 137.

sufficient to denote the achromatic colours of everyday life. We shall not discuss here any further the principle of economy in the creation of words, but presumably we should not have so few designations for greys unless the qualities themselves denoted by one word represented a natural and distinct grouping. These five qualities from the black-white series are selected to characterize the achromatic colours ; they also have a special rôle in the recognition of colours. If an observer sees upon a disc A a certain colour which he is to equate in quality to a colour on disc B, he frequently endeavours first of all to characterize the more distant colour, usually in verbal form.[1] The observer finds himself forced to this procedure by the particular experimental conditions. The difference between the illuminations of discs A and B forces him to a great extent to consider the *quality* of the colours, while in the case of colours seen under the *same* conditions of illumination, judgment is passed upon qualitative *difference* rather than upon qualities themselves. Thus the observer says something like this : I see the colour of disc A as white, grey, etc., and will vary the colour of disc B until the same name may be applied to it. If it were true to say that under the conditions of illumination obtaining here the recognition of " white," " light grey," " middle grey," etc., varies in difficulty according to the colour seen, we should be able to understand the saltatory character of our curves. It is actually true that in the production of a scale of achromatic colours the observer naturally tends to resort to a grouping of the various members similar to that expressed in our curves. When I gave observers L and N this problem, it was striking how easily they discharged the task. This justifies the assumption that the observers were not deceiving themselves in what they said about the process of comparison. It was most natural for these observers to distinguish only *four* qualities in forming groups.

[1] *Cf.* the rôle played by linguistic characterization of colours in the comparison of colours separated by temporal intervals. Frank Angell, *Wundts Philos. Stud.*, 1902, 19.

The following values were chosen on disc *B* :

	Observer L	Observer N
White . .	360°–135° *W*	360°–210° *W*
Light grey .	135°– 42° *W*	210°– 70° *W*
Dark grey .	42°– 5° *W*	70°– 20° *W*
Black . .	5°– 0° *W*	20°– 0° *W*

The values for disc *A* were these :

	Observer L	Observer N
White . .	360°–203° *W*	360°–234° *W*
Light grey .	203°–140° *W*	234°–110° *W*
Dark grey .	140°– 20° *W*	110°– 19° *W*
Black . .	20°– 0° *W*	19°– 0° *W*

Now are there any relationships between the irregularities of the curves and these values ? In the present context, the values on disc *A* are most important. The observer starts from these values, considered as stable, in the process of comparison. It is sufficient to determine that, as we expected, the observers distinguished four groups. I should like to add that subjectively it is easiest for the observers to separate the first group from the others. We may draw this conclusion : It is probable that in judging colours the observers place them in certain groups (such as white, light gey, dark grey and black) and that for some reason, hard to formulate any more exactly now, the various groups differ in the ease with which they are recognized (white being the easiest, black the hardest) when the intensity of illumination is reduced.

One of Gelb's patients saw steps—four to be exact—when he was looking at the black-white series in front of him. It seems very probable that there is an inner relationship between this fact and the division into four groups such as we have found. Gelb himself seems to have overlooked the analogy.

Let us try to compare the qualities distinguishable on discs *A* and *B*. All colours obtained by settings from 21° to 360° upon disc *A* for observer *L* may be produced

upon disc *B* with much less variation. We have represented graphically in Fig. 3 the correlation of the settings
upon *A* and *B*. *L* required only the settings from 222·3°
to about 6° *W* on *B*. Here we must note, of course, that
strictly speaking the black qualities which may be obtained
upon *A* through variation from 6° to 21° *W* are absent
on *B*. The enrichment undergone by the colours on *A*
through this variation is so significant that even this
result shows a greater wealth in distinguishable colours
upon *B* as compared with those appearing upon *A* when
the white component is varied from 6° to 360°.

We might also raise here the question as to what
qualitative changes are undergone by the continuum of

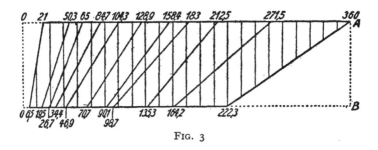

FIG. 3

achromatic surface colours when we present them under
the conditions prevailing in the case of *A* instead of
under the "normal" conditions of illumination of *B*.
In the illustration (Fig. 4) we give the above determined
qualitative judgments of observer *L*. Since these groupings grew out of absolute qualitative judgments and not
out of comparisons, they give also a picture of the qualitatively different groups which we must ordinarily assume
for achromatic surface colours standing under conditions
of illumination like those of disc *A*.

In the figure two equally long parallel lines indicate
the sectors upon *A* and *B* which may be set as white. I
have marked on these two lines the points which bound
the four qualitatively demarcated regions. The distance
between the lines symbolizes the distance from *A* to *B*

(about 2·5 m.) in our experiments. If the distance r–s represents all the settings on B which may be designated as " white " and t–u the corresponding settings upon A, then the area r–s–t–u symbolizes all the colours called " white " which we may get as we pass gradually from the intensity of illumination of B to that of A. We still have to determine whether we may assume that the line connecting r with t is really straight, as we have drawn it for the sake of simplicity. With the intensities of illumination which we used, it is certainly true that the quality white occupies greater space upon B than upon A. If we pass beyond the limits (135°, 203°) by the same number of steps, we come to the boundary of the " light grey " region sooner for A than for B. The relationship

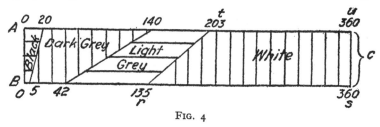

FIG. 4

is exactly opposite as regards " dark grey " and " black." Whereas for B the colour extends as white over a broad range, and passes through numerous light grey steps into dark grey, upon A the dark grey is particularly broad (with a narrow band of black at one end), and is considerably closer to the white. The relationships found here may be realized clearly if we use two scales of eighteen members as described above (p. 79) or better still, Burzlaff's scale of forty-eight members. If we place the one scale in the neighbourhood of disc A and the other in the neighbourhood of disc B, we see very well that the white and light grey qualities occupy a much greater region upon B than upon A. On the other hand, the dark grey colours upon the farther scale occupy a broader range and are not as far removed from the white. We may observe in pen-and-ink drawings or in copper engravings that the colours which, in normal illumination, form a transitional region between black and white, recede when the intensity of illumination is strongly reduced and the white and dark grey tones come more closely together. This observation is also confirmed by an attentive inspection of pictures in which a low intensity of illumination is portrayed, *e.g.*, in pictures of moonlit landscapes. In many of his fantastic compositions aiming at an impression of reduced illumination or of twilight, A. Kubin has used the principle of the grouping of brightness-values which appeared in our observations.

§ 20. Episcotister Experiments

We used the following set-up in a number of different experiments. A schematic drawing may make it clear (Fig. 5). At a distance of 90 cm. from the middle window W_2 of the experimental room a black screen *s* was set up, and in this two circular holes, a_1 and a_2, with diameters of 0·7 cm. were cut. The distance between them was 3 cm. At a distance of 1·4 m. from this screen were two discs, B_1 and B_2, each with a diameter of about 11 cm. B_1 stood against a screen D_1 (diameter 20 cm.) whose brightness was variable, and which served as its background. Similarly a neutral grey screen D_2 served as background for B_2. Approximately ½ cm. behind the opening a_2 of the screen *s* was a variable episcotister covered with velvet black. This was so set up that an eye near its margin could look through it at B_2. In the experiments the observer kept his eye so close to *s* that practically no light passed through a_2 to the rotating episcotister disc. Since the episcotister was covered with

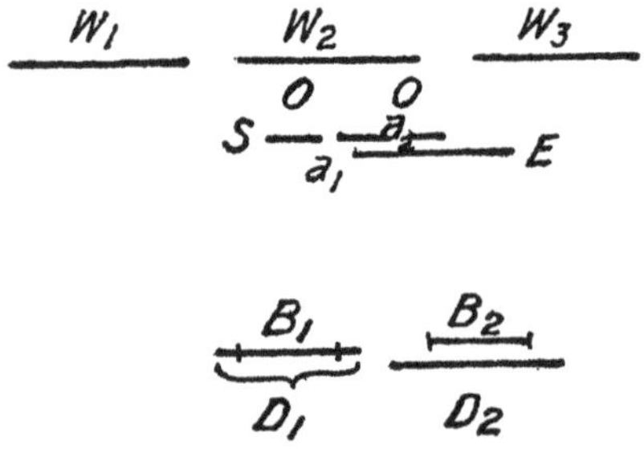

FIG. 5

black, and received only small quantities of light from the other side, we may for all practical purposes *neglect* the amount of light falling directly from the episcotister disc itself into the observer's eye.

We performed certain experiments in which the opening of the episcotister was varied. B_2 was a disc of 360° W. When the observer looked through a_2, he saw B_2 with its surroundings quite clearly. Now the problem was this : with a given opening of the episcotister (*e.g.*, 3°), the observer was to set up a colour of the same quality on disc B_1, which was seen through a_1. B_1 was varied in accordance with the method of limits. The backgrounds of B_2 and B_1 were equated as nearly as possible in their retinal effects, so that the effect of the background of B_2 was determined according to Talbot's law by the light-intensity of S_2 and the opening of the episcotister at the same time. We used this procedure to get approximately equal contrast conditions for the two discs ; in this arrangement the same contrast relations are present if we assume that contrast effects are determined essentially by relationships between retinal excitations.

RESULTS FOR OBSERVER P

$$B_2 = 360° W. \quad n = 8.$$
$$E\ 90°.[1] \quad B_1 = 117° W \quad E\ 10°. \quad B_1 = 87° W$$
$$E\ 30°. \quad B_1 = \ 98° W \quad E\ 3°. \quad B_1 = 81° W$$

If the brightness impressions brought about by our stimulus combination $(E + B_2)$ [2] were determined only by Talbot's law, the settings on B_1 would have been quite different from those actually obtained. For E 90°, for example, a setting of 90° W on B_1 would be too bright, since as we have shown, the light reflected from the velvet black of E (although not that from the velvet black of B_1) may be neglected. Therefore our settings deviate

---

[1] E 90°, E 30°, etc., mean that the episcotister disc had a sector of 90°, 30°, etc.
[2] We use $(E + B_2)$ as a short symbol for the stimulus-combination made up of the episcotister and the disc B_2.

by more than 27° W from what we should expect. The smaller the opening of the episcotister becomes, the more the results differ from our expectations; indeed, with E 3°, the difference reaches a surprising magnitude, more than 81°–3°. We cannot draw from our results any objections against Talbot's law in the case of the situation $(E + B_2)$ unless our equations are perfect *in every respect*. That is not, however, the case. These are equations in *quality*, but the settings upon B_1 all have a higher degree of *insistence*. In this connection we note the interesting fact that with settings of 117°, 98°, 87° and 82° W, we obtain upon B_2 four different light greys corresponding to four qualitatively equal impressions of lower insistence and pronouncedness. The distinctness of this difference in insistence between the qualities in question increases noticeably from E 90° to E 3°. With a larger opening of the episcotister than we used, we arrive at qualities resembling white more closely, but the distinctness of the difference in pronouncedness also recedes.

It is easier to present our results if we interpret our experiments as if the observer, while looking at B_2, were " taking into account " the reduction in the intensity of illumination brought about by the episcotister. We note, first of all, that this is not *ideal*, for in that case all the settings upon B_2 would have to be 360° W. The qualitative change in the colour of B_2, *i.e.*, its shift toward grey, becomes absolutely greater as the opening of the episcotister is made smaller, and B_2 approximates grey more and more as the corresponding value of $(E + B_2)$, calculated according to Talbot's law, becomes weaker. The B-quotients (B-series) in our experiments are as follows :

E 90°.   121·0 : 360 = 0·33 E 10°.   91·6 : 360 = 0·24
E 30°.   102·4 : 360 = 0·28 E 3°.   85·7 : 360 = 0·23

All these B-quotients appear to be rather low when we compare them with those obtained in the other experiments (with $A = 360° W$) (p. 97 ff.). This means that here the " taking into account " of the particular conditions of illumination approaches the ideal less than in earlier experiments. The brightness quotient for E 90° is absolutely greater than that for E 30°. We find quite a different state of affairs when we compare in terms of their action upon the retina the light-intensities of B_1 and the corresponding values $(E + B_2)$. Then we obtain these values (Q-quotients):

E 90°.   121·0 : 90 = 1·34 E 10°.   91·6 : 10 = 9·16
E 30°.   102·4 : 30 = 3·41 E 3°.   85·7 : 3 = 28·6

It follows from these values that if we consider the *physiological intensities* in the case of E 90°, E 30°, E 10° and E 3°, the brightening undergone by B_2 increases considerably from E 90° to E 3°. There is a slight brightening even for E 90°, but it is surprisingly high for E 3°.

The episcotister brings about a reduction in the intensity of the illumination of the entire visual field similar to that appearing in natural twilight. If, as in our experiments described on p. 95 ff., we observe the wall in the background of a room, with the objects on it or near it, a reduced intensity of illumination prevails in almost the entire visual field or at least in a large part of it. Thus there is no essential difference between the reducing of the illumination of normally illuminated objects by means of an episcotister and that induced by placing objects in the back part of a room. We can combine the experiments on illumination perspective with the episcotister experiments by observing our arrangement for illumination perspective sometimes directly and at other times through the episcotister. The effect upon illumination is then as if the daylight illumination in the room were being reduced. The striking thing about illumination perspective is that we see side by side in the visual field objects with different degrees of illumination which decrease regularly with distance from the light-source, and that we either apprehend them simultaneously or at least can turn from one to another in quick succession.

§ 21. The Insistence of Achromatic Colours

We shall call that one of two colours the more "insistent" which seems to possess the power of catching the eye more readily and of holding it more steadily. In general, if two achromatic colours are seen in the same illumination and against the same background, the brighter will be of this nature.[1] Now how do matters stand as regards the insistence of achromatic colours when the intensity of illumination is changed? The following experiments deal with this question.

In the experiments described in the preceding sections, B_1 always surpassed B_2 in insistence. I asked one observer to equate the two discs in insistence. According to his reports, the observer was able to adopt two attitudes. He could, on the one hand, observe how the discs *stood out from their backgrounds*, and on the other hand set the discs in such a way that he felt himself *gripped to an equal extent* by the two. I asked him to observe this latter process, since it occurred to me to test under what conditions individual colours (not colour-distances or degrees of relief) act equally upon the observer. I hardly need to say expressly that the following insistence-equations are *qualitative inequalities*, B_1 being distinctly darker in all cases :

$B_2 = 360° W.$
$$E\ 30°.\quad B_1 = 25° W \qquad\qquad E3°.\quad B_1 = 1° W$$
$$E\ 10°.\quad B_1 = 9° W$$

We may now compare with each other the light-intensities which we must assume as effective for the retina in these insistence equations of B_1 and B_2. Having corrected for the white-valence of the black of B_1, we obtain the following values :

$$E\ 30°.\quad B_1 = 30·7° W,\ B_2 = 30° W$$
$$E\ 10°.\quad B_1 = 14·8° W,\ B_2 = 10° W$$
$$E\ \ 3°.\quad B_1 = 7·0° W,\ B_2 = 3° W$$

---

[1] " Insistence is not built up secondarily upon simple experiences of brightness, but is itself the more primitive experience." Insistence means " the dimension of the experienced effects upon the self." Metzger, p. 22.

We see that the values of B_1 and B_2 do not differ very much from each other in the two situations. The values of B_1 are somewhat larger, and when the opening of the episcotister is made smaller, the difference between the values of B_1 and B_2 increases. Two achromatic surface colours appear equally insistent, in spite of their qualitative difference, when the disc seen through the episcotister is approximately equal in retinal effect to the other disc. Later we shall refer frequently to this theoretically important result.

In connection with these experiments, I shall report some observations dealing with the same question under the experimental conditions described in § 19. In those experiments on illumination perspective, the settings upon B appeared more insistent than those upon A under all conditions. I attempted now to discover for two particular values of A equally insistent settings of B. I instructed the observers to apprehend the surface colour of each disc by itself, and to compare their insistences. Without such an instruction, the observer is so set from the start that he sees both discs under conditions which are as *similar* as he can make them, *e.g.*, he localizes both on the wall or perhaps in a *fictitious* plane before the wall. That would naturally introduce into the experiments an entirely new factor, a levelling of the conditions of illumination of A and B, and this must be excluded here.

OBSERVER B

Method of Limits. $n = 4$

I. Equation for quality.
    1. Disc A : 360° W Disc B : 183·5° W
    2. Disc A : 180° W Disc B : 69·4° W

II. Equation for insistence.
    1. Disc A : 360° W Disc B : 118·4° W
    2. Disc A : 180° W Disc B : 57·5° W

III. Equation with reduction-screen.
    1. Disc A : 360° W Disc B : 104·4° W
    2. Disc A : 180° W Disc B : 51·3° W

In these experiments we are concerned with a comparison of the values in II with those in I and III. Let us select first the values for $A = 360° W$. The value in II differs quite considerably from that in I and closely approaches that in III. The respective differences are $65\cdot1° W$ and $14\cdot0° W$. The conclusion is that an equation made after reduction stands closer to an equation for insistence than to an equation for quality. I even suspect that the values in II and III would have approached identity still more if the observer had made his judgment even more than he really did in terms of insistence alone. Naturally it is not very easy to equate discs A and B simply in terms of their insistence. Therefore any great and obtrusive qualitative difference between A and B must affect the settings in such a way that the difference between the values of II and III is positive, as we found in our experiments. When settings for equal insistence are made, disc A appears white or light grey and disc B varies from white to dark grey. If secondary comparisons were not involved, the difference between the values of II and III would certainly be smaller. We may perhaps note a certain confirmation of this hypothesis in the results of the experiments with $A = 180° W$, in which the difference between the values of II and III amounts to only $6\cdot2° W$. When $A = 180° W$, the qualitative difference between discs A and B is not nearly as great as in experiments with $A = 360° W$.[1] The present data supplement the result already obtained in the episcotister experiments : *In experiments on illumination perspective, two colours under different conditions of illumination appear equally insistent when they reflect approximately the same amounts of light into the eye.*

On account of its theoretical significance, I have also carried out experiments on the problem of insistence with shadowed colours. For the sake of coherence I shall report the results here. In these new experiments the procedure was indirect, in that I was trying to determine how much the light upon two differently illuminated

[1] *Cf.* p. 98 f.

surface colours must be increased for this increase to be noted. If the *same increase* of light is necessary for two differently illuminated surface colours reflecting light of equal retinal effect, then it is very probable that we may ascribe the same intensity to the psychophysical excitations corresponding to the two impressions. The experimental situation has also a more general applicability in other cases in which the limens of colours are to be determined.

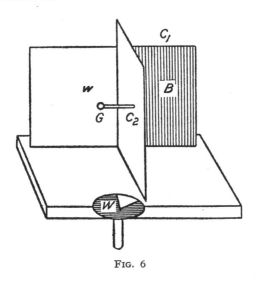

FIG. 6

A rectangular card C_1 about 40 cm. high and 60 cm. wide was covered half with white (w) and half with black (b) paper. In front of this card, which was placed in a vertical position, I set up perpendicular to it and touching it, a white card C_2 which threw its shadow over the entire white surface. When the window-shutters were partially closed, the illumination in the experimental room was reduced to such a point that under reduction the black and white papers matched; therefore they must have had the same retinal effect. Under direct inspection, they naturally appear quite different from each other in quality, the right being deep black and the left a colour lying between light grey and grey. Now, in the following way, we increased the retinal excitations, observing the papers directly. A round cover-glass (*G*), such as is used in microscopic work, 10 mm. in diameter and 0·14 mm. thick, was fixed upon a cardboard strip about ½ mm. thick by means of a drop of glue, and was attached to the card C_2 about 10 cm. in front of and parallel to the white surface, as may be seen from the figure. This cover-glass absorbed a certain amount of the light reflected from *w*; therefore to an observer looking from the front at the shaded surface it appeared darker than its surroundings, unless there were, *under* and *in front of* the small glass, objects which reflected through the glass to the observer's eye an amount of light equal to or greater than that absorbed by the glass. In the first case, the cover-glass becomes altogether invisible; in the latter case, it appears brighter than its surroundings. Now I set in this region a colour-wheel *W* with a horizontal surface, whose light might be reflected by the cover-glass into the observer's eye. We found upon the colour-wheel a brightness which caused the entire area of the cover-glass to stand out as *just distinguishable* from its surroundings, *i.e.*, from the coloured surface lying behind it. First we determined the limen for the shadowed white paper by means of the method of limits. The observations were monocular, in order that there should be no double images of the cover-glass when C_1 was fixated. For the determination of the corresponding limen for the un-shadowed and approximately normally illuminated black, the conditions as regards the reflection of light from the cover-glass should be the same; therefore I moved the screen C_1 somewhat back and to the side, until the black part of C_1 lay behind the cover-glass. I convinced myself, by making a brightness-equation after reduction, that the amount of light reflected by the black paper suffered no change through this displacement. It now appeared that the same increase of light was necessary in the two cases to make the brightening noticeable. Sometimes white and sometimes black required a somewhat higher value in the settings. The same increases in light were noted subjectively in the *same way*, *i.e.*, in both cases the cover-glass stood out as *just distinguishable* from its background.   Naturally these two areas did not give an impression of full equality in colour, for the increase in light upon the light grey appeared as a still lighter grey and upon the black as a dark grey.   The observers agreed that the field *w* appeared somewhat different when they did not, as usual, let their eyes rove over it freely but, as here, attempted to determine the limen exactly.   In this case the perceived light grey underwent a slight shift toward a somewhat darker grey.   We shall discuss below (§ 33) the receding of colour-constancy when a more or less critical attitude is adopted, as noted in this observation.[1] Since we know that colour-constancy under reduced illumination is relatively strongest for *white*, it was unnecessary to repeat our experiments with other qualities.   We also performed some experiments in which the white paper was shadowed in different degrees (but less strongly than in the first experiment), and in which the black paper was replaced by grey papers which were, under reduction, equal to the variously illuminated white papers.   The limens for any two colours of the same pair were approximately the same.   From these results it seems possible to draw the following conclusion :   If surface colours provide the same retinal excitation, equal peripheral increases in light are always necessary to be just noticeable, regardless of the impressions which the colours make before reduction.   We shall call this the *law of the conservation of the total psychophysical intensity of retinal excitations*.   This law is subject to limitations when configural factors, *e.g.*, those involving the difference between figure and ground, become effective.   After Rubin [2] had noted that figure and ground are adaptable to illumination in different degrees, Gelb and Granit showed that the limen for figure is higher than that for ground.[3]   Aside from such limitations, our generalization

---

[1] Monocular fixation likewise caused colour-constancy to decrease to some extent. *Cf.* § 34.

[2] *Op. cit.*, p. 56.   [3] *Zsch. f. Psychol.*, 1923, 93.

H

would seem to be valid. Gelb himself assents to it, since he occasionally utilizes it in his writings.[1] In this connection I should like to cite certain results obtained recently by Metzger in the so-called total field.[2] He found that a total field with a brightness value of 12 is just as insistent as a small field with a brightness value of 10,000 ; the total field is thus just as insistent as a small field 830 times as bright. A calculation made on the basis of certain plausible assumptions leads Metzger to suspect that under the simple conditions of his experiment, " the impression is proportional to the total amount of energy involved." [3]

§ 22. ILLUMINATION AND THE DIFFERENTIAL LIMEN

The experiments described above already suggest an answer to the question concerning our differential sensitivity for achromatic surface colours under various intensities of illumination. Let us consider a series of whites differing in pronouncedness. What change of intensity must whites *of different degrees of pronouncedness undergo* if an increase or decrease in brightness is to be brought about ? We may formulate as follows the principle of the conservation of total psychophysical intensity : The differential limen for colours of different pronouncedness depends only upon the position of the colours in the black-white series *after they are reduced to the same illumination.* After reduction to the *same* illumination, the different degrees of pronouncedness of

---

[1] Gelb remarks, in regard to Hering's familiar shadow-experiment, that " in the shift from weakly illuminated white to strongly illuminated black something remains invariant, *viz.*, the degree of liveliness or insistence of the disc. This may be explained in terms of the fact that the same amount of light reaches the eye from the rotating disc both before and after the shift ; we know, however, that the degree of insistence of a coloured surface depends only upon the intensity of retinal excitation (Katz)." Gelb, p. 674 f.

[2] Total field (*Ganzfeld*) refers to that state in which the whole visual field is uniformly coloured, uniformly structured and uniformly illuminated. Metzger's observations were made with an apparatus described in *Psychol. Forsch.*, 1929, 13.

[3] Metzger, I, p. 23.

white fall at different points in the black-white series corresponding to this illumination ; hence it is unquestionable that the liminal values we are seeking should be different. From our experimental results we may deduce the following principle : *Differential sensitivity for achromatic surface colours under illuminations of different intensities follows the same laws as does differential sensitivity for these colours when they are reduced to the same illumination.*

We may supplement this generalization in the following way. When a certain stimulus situation is bounded by two light stimuli of any intensity, the sensory fields corresponding to this stimulus situation may vary as a result of totality factors which affect vision ; but the *same* number of *just noticeable* differences must be distinguishable within each of these different sensory fields. The following principle has been formulated by Marzynski to cover this fact : " Both a just noticeable and a very distinctly noticeable difference may correspond to the same stimulus difference."[1]

In connection with the principle formulated above (p. 113), we may mention one of Jaensch's observations, which assumes significance only in the light of what we have been reporting here. After Jaensch had confirmed in micropsy experiments the observations by W. Koster and others of certain apparent changes in the brightness of achromatic colours (brightening of bright colours, darkening of dark colours), he asked how the differential limen for achromatic colours behaves in artificial micropsy and macropsy. Since a certain brightness difference appeared greater in micropsy than without it, it seemed obvious to expect a higher differential limen for the latter. This expectation was *not*, however, confirmed. " We may summarize the results by saying that the differential limen is certainly no lower in micropsy."[2] What does this mean except that our principle, as given

[1] *Zsch. f. Psychol.*, 1927, 87.
[2] E. R. Jaensch, *Zur Analyse der Gesichtswahrnehmungen.* Leipzig, 1909, p. 146.

above, may be extended even to these colour-impressions observed in micropsy experiments ?

Let us spend a moment in describing the colour-phenomena which Jaensch observed in these micropsy experiments. Although in micropsy there was a very distinct change of the surface colours, all of them appearing to be more strongly illuminated, it was still "quite impossible" to make an equation between the surface colours before and during the micropsy. In the light of these results, we can hardly doubt that here we have achromatic surface colours which differ in pronouncedness and between which no perfect equation is possible. Further observations by Koster and Jaensch provide evidence favouring our assumption that we have here relationships between illumination and illuminated object. There were great *individual* differences in the distinctness with which the various observers perceived the colour-changes in micropsy, and also (according to Jaensch) the phenomena displayed, at least in direct vision, a high degree of lability. We also found these two tendencies in our experiments ; we have already mentioned individual differences and shall return later (§ 33) to the lability of the phenomena. Finally, the great importance of indirect vision for the phenomena we have mentioned, as emphasized by Jaensch, also implies that relationships between illumination and illuminated object were involved. We shall discuss later (Chapter III) the significance of the retinal periphery for the perception of illumination.

§ 23. Weber's Law and the Episcotister

We might go to Weber's law for an explanation of our episcotister experiments, for this law is held to be approximately valid as a basis for the recognition of colours seen in illumination of various intensities. Yet this would not be justified, for aside from other points, Weber's law does not take full cognizance of the phenomenological state of affairs which we have when illumination is changed. If the intensity of illumination changes, the relative differences in light-intensity between adjacent surfaces remain equally great, and this, according to Weber's law, is synonymous with " equally noticeable." According to Weber's law, differences between achromatic colours remain equally noticeable when illumination is reduced. Thus, on a copper engraving with all conceivable gradations from white to black, the contours should remain even when it is seen through an episcotister with a very small opening, and hence the form represented in the engraving should be recognizable. That does not explain, however, why the achromatic *colour surfaces themselves* are also apprehended in approximately their own colours—white as white, light grey as light grey, etc.—under widely varying conditions of illumination. When we read the accounts of the significance of Weber's law for the recognition of colours under varied illumination, we miss references to the changes which colours undergo when illumination is changed. Every change in illumination intensity also brings about a *qualitative* change in achromatic surface colours. Under these conditions the qualitative change may be very slight; but in most cases there is a change in *pronouncedness.* Thus we may recognize a colour as a white which has been only slightly modified, although its insistence has become quite different. Therefore Weber's law is not sufficient to explain our results. In so far as it contributes to the perception of objects through the conservation of their contours, we might appeal to it (in addition to boundary contrast) as *one* factor explaining our episcotister experiments. We shall appreciate later how important the preservation of contours is for colour-constancy. Here we may simply point out that Weber's law does not, as has sometimes been assumed, explain the recognition of colours under change of illumination.

In the work cited above (p. 115), Marzynski has studied in detail the relations between Weber's law and colour-constancy. He found a constancy of differential sensitivity only when the light-intensity was changed by means of a change in illumination and when phenomena of colour-constancy played a rôle. "We were never able to discover any constancy of differential sensitivity in those experiments in which transformation played no rôle."

§ 24. QUALITY FLICKER AND ILLUMINATION FLICKER

When Maxwell discs are rotated not quite rapidly enough to produce fusion, the familiar phenomenon of flicker appears. This flicker differs markedly from that which may be observed in the case of a combination $(E+B)$.[1] In the case of the discs, we see the flicker at that position in space at which the colours are located. We really see the colour itself flickering. In the restless confusion of bright and dark, there is to a certain extent no point capable of holding fixation, and not even the smallest particles of the surface are at rest. The flicker which we observe when we are looking at a surface colour through an episcotister is of quite a different sort. In a certain way it stands out from the disc itself. It might be better to say that there is a flickering *across* the disc or *before* it in space than to say that the disc *itself* observed through the episcotister is flickering. The flickering slips over the disc much as lights and shadows slip over surface colours. These light patterns are not perceived as really belonging to the colour of the disc itself. While in the case of Maxwell discs *everything is in movement*, the surface seen through the episcotister appears at rest behind the flicker. To distinguish these two types of flicker, Bühler [2] has coined the terms "quality flicker" and "illumination flicker" which characterize strikingly their phenomenal difference. The resting state of the surface behind the episcotister is particularly distinct at its edge, where the disc is sharply distinguished from the background, as well as at the knob of the electric wheel, whose contour is sharply demarcated from the disc. Even if Maxwell discs are very well cut and centred, their boundaries never stand out as sharply from the background when they are

---

[1] *Cf.* p. 105.   [2] Bühler, p. 120.

rotated as when they are stationary, and the contour of the knob of the wheel always seems blurred when it is moving. The quality flicker of Maxwell discs decreases gradually as the speed of rotation is increased, although its character is not essentially changed. In the case of the combination $(E + B)$, the illumination flicker is somewhat changed in type under these circumstances. When the flicker is weak, the points which are apprehended more acutely stand out distinctly. They seem to be completely at rest, no flicker being perceptible in front of them, while the flicker is still perfectly distinct in front of their surroundings. Through this close fixation the minute details of the grain of the paper become distinctly visible. If we permit the eye to rove here and there over the disc, a flickerless region accompanies it.[1] I agree with Bühler when he considers the emergence of micromorphic details not as the effect but as the cause of lack of flicker.[2] On rotating Maxwell discs flickering also becomes somewhat less prominent when a particular point is sharply fixated, but the decrease is certainly not as marked as it is under the same condition in the case of $(E + B)$. In the fusion of periodic lights when an episcotister is used, there is accordingly a certain difference between the behaviour of central and that of peripheral parts of the retina, a difference which cannot be observed in the same degree if Maxwell discs are used. To explain this difference we might think of physiological factors, especially of the superiority of certain parts of the retina over its peripheral parts in perception of macrostructures and microstructures. On account of its proximity, the edge of the episcotister can be projected upon the retina only in dispersion circles. Thus it does not make a sharp

---

[1] Metzger describes the "twitching" which appears when a supplementary light stimulus is introduced into or removed from the total field. "For the unprejudiced observer, it includes the entire surface; but if we look at a particular point to see what is happening there, the twitching is seen as before as including the entire surface. But it is impossible to say whether anything else is going on at the point observed. Sometimes there is distinct twitching everywhere except at the *region of fixation.*" W. Metzger, I, p. 27.

[2] Bühler, p. 120.

contour upon the retina, as is the case with the boundary contour between the black and white sectors of a Maxwell disc. Since the difference between central and peripheral vision is not nearly as great with respect to sensitivity to movement as with respect to visual acuity, it is of less significance for the periphery than for the centre of the retina whether a sharp or blurred contour is passing over it. It probably makes little difference for the periphery whether it fuses periodic lights delivered from a Maxwell disc or lights from the combination $(E+B)$. Thus the distinction between quality flickers and illumination flickers is not substantiated for isolated parts of the retinal periphery, if they are not too extensive. The vague contour of the episcotister still permits us, even during the flickering, to apprehend form elements at the highly acute centre of the retina. The legibility of printing seen through an episcotister and lying in the position of B is scarcely reduced even by a strong flicker, since the contours are strengthened by contrast and preserved with astonishing tenacity. There are really, in a strict sense, no " contour flickers," but only flickers referred either to colour-matter (quality flickers) or to illumination (illumination flickers). There may appear at the contours changes in position or in configuration which, if they are rhythmical, we often call oscillations. Even in their quantitative aspects, these oscillations are subject to a law which is different from that for flicker ; in his experiments on geometric optical illusions, in which by the addition of lines the effects might be produced or destroyed at will, Wingender has shown that " the inertia of the apparatus which apprehends changes in form is considerably greater than (about ten times as great as) that of the sensory organs, as laid down in Talbot's law."[1]

Flicker is a sign that a rapidly oscillating process is going on at a point in the nervous centres involved in the act of vision. Let us contrast the agreement in the phenomena of flicker and fusion with the great difference

[1] *Zsch. f. Psychol.*, 1919, 82.

in quality and pronouncedness of the colour-phenomena observed under the same stimulus-conditions as we have described above.[1] If we do so, we are unable to resist the impression that phenomena of flicker depend primarily upon the intensity and composition of the light-waves impinging upon the external eye and the resulting peripheral excitations, and on the other hand are essentially independent of central conditions. This fact represents a welcome supplement to our discussions in § 22. We may conclude that the intensity of the psychophysical processes mediated by centripetal excitation depends only upon the intensities of retinal excitation. This shows that *the conditions under which these processes arise from the fusion of periodic retinal excitations are quite similar.*

Th. Haack has recently reported experiments on contrast flicker, *i.e.*, on flicker which is induced in an objectively constant field by neighbouring flickers; she was able to demonstrate that the two forms distinguished above—quality flicker and illumination flicker—appear even under these conditions. She was also able to show that contrast flicker is strongly inhibited by effects originating in macrostructure and microstructure.[2]

§ 25. Surface Colours in Light and Shadow

Two colour-wheels, B_1 and B_2, were set up at a short distance from each other. They received light through a window at the side of the experimental room. Between the two wheels was a device which permitted us to fix at this place a sheet of paper, the translucency of which might be varied. This made it possible to vary within certain wide limits the amount of light falling upon B_2 and hence to produce upon it a shadow varying in darkness. B_1 and B_2 were observed either directly or after reduction, and a neutral grey cloth served as their background.

We performed experiments with four shadows of

---

[1] *Cf*. p. 105 ff.
[2] Theodora Haack, " Kontrast und Transformation," *Zsch. f. Psychol.*, 1929, 112.

different depths. B_2 was placed in the shadow of a black cardboard disc (A-experiments), of a surface made of folded tissue-paper (B-experiments), of a surface made of single-ply tissue-paper (C-experiments), or of a surface made of oiled tissue-paper (D-experiments). The photographs of our apparatus given in § 26 may assist in showing to what extent not only the colour on B_2 but also the visible parts of the wheel and its surroundings were included in the shadow. We always used a disc of 360° W for B_2. We found as follows a pair of values for each particular shadowing. After a reduction screen had been lowered, we established a perfect equation between the two reduced colours by changing B_1 according to the method of limits. After determining the value under reduction (Value I), we raised the screen and had the observers look at the disc in such a way that they were able to survey completely the conditions of illumination. The equation between the reduced colours was *never* accepted under these new conditions, the shadowed disc always appearing too whitish. The setting on B_1 was changed until the observer reported that the colours on the two wheels were equal in quality (Value II). In this experiment we encountered a difficulty which had not appeared in our earlier experiments on surface colours in different intensities of illumination. When the observer tried to abstract from the shadowing of B_2, the quality of the colour itself seemed to vary significantly as his attitude changed, even though the external conditions remained the same. Its quality varied *according to the degree to which the observer became " absorbed " in looking at it*. Since this " absorption " seemed to depend upon the exposition-time, I chose a *constant* period of about 3 sec. for establishing Values II, the two colours being exposed by means of a curtain hung in front of the reduction screen. This length of time was quite sufficient for the observer to make his comparison. The influence of the exposition-time was also studied in its own right.[1] The time for the " reduced " setting (Values

---

[1] *Cf.* § 29.

I) was left to the discretion of the observers. This was also the case in the earlier experiments on illumination perspective and those with the episcotister, where the exposition-time is certainly not without some significance but does not have as great an influence as in the present experiments. B_2 presents decidedly the more interesting colour ; the attitude of the observer toward it might well be called " active," for he tried to *penetrate into its quality*. The observer tended to let B_1 act upon him ; *he resigned himself to the impression* and looked at it only casually. Therefore, in general, only a small fraction of the entire exposition-time was devoted to B_1.

OBSERVER R

Disc $B_2 = 360°$ W. $n = 8$

A-experiments
     Value I.   Disc $B_1 = $ 4·2° W. Mean variation 2·4°
     „ II.   „ $B_1 = 116·0°$ W. „ „ 19·2°

B-experiments
     Value I.   „ $B_1 = $ 65·9° W. „ „ 3·3°
     „ II.   „ $B_1 = 178·6°$ W. „ „ 11·3°

C-experiments
     Value I.   „ $B_1 = $ 80·1° W. „ „ 6·1°
     „ II.   „ $B_1 = 180·0°$ W. „ „ 17·1°

D-experiments
     Value I.   „ $B_1 = 202·4°$ W. „ „ 10·6°
     „ II.   „ $B_1 = 246·0°$ W. „ „ 15·5°

We began the C and D experiments somewhat later than the A and B experiments. This explains the fact that Value II of the C experiments (180·0° W) was lower than we should expect from the corresponding Value I and from the Values II of the A and B experiments. In general, the brightening tends to decrease somewhat in the course of the experiments.

If the shadowing of B_2 had been completely taken into account, all of the settings for Values II would have been 360° W ; the settings which we really found, however, lay far below this. In order to see to what extent the shadow was only partially taken into account, let us form, as before, the brightness quotients of the B-series. We find the following series of values : 0·33, 0·50, 0·50, and 0·69. We may draw this conclusion : *The qualitative modification of a white disc lying in a shadow becomes greater as the shadow is intensified.* Our results give a decidedly different picture if we take account of the light-intensities issuing from the shadowed colours and the brightnesses with which they are perceived. The brightening undergone by the colours under shadows of different degrees of intensity may then be expressed in terms of the following series of quotients of Values I and II : 11·8, 2·6, 2·2, and 1·2 (Q-series). We see from this series that *the deeper the shadow is, the greater is the relative brightening of a white surface seen in it.* The value for the A experiments may be considered extraordinarily high.

OBSERVER U

Disc $B_2 = 360°$ $W.$ $n = 8$

A-experiments
  Value I.   Disc $B_1 =$ 8·3° $W.$ Mean variation   3·9°
    „   II.   „ $B_1 =$ 97·7° $W.$ „   „   11·7°

C-experiments
  Value I.   „ $B_1 =$ 51·0° $W.$ „   „   4·6°
    „   II.   „ $B_1 =$ 156·2° $W.$ „   „   19·6°

D-experiments
  Value I.   „ $B_1 =$ 71·9° $W.$ „   „   3·6°
    „   II.   „ $B_1 =$ 166·5° $W.$ „   „   18·4°

In this case, as before, we form the quotients of the B-series and find these values : 0·28, 0·45, and 0·47. This series confirms the generalization formulated above on this page.

We obtain the following values for the Q-series : 7·1, 2·9, and 2·2. This series gives a picture quite similar to the corresponding series of observer R.

In establishing Values II, the observers were about

80 cm. from the two discs. The brightening of disc B_2 was less when it was observed from a greater distance.

We obtained the following results for observer R, for example, when the distance was 3 m., the other conditions being the same as before :

A-experiments
    Value II.   Disc $B_1 = 15\cdot0°$ W.   Mean variation $6\cdot2°$

B-experiments
    Value II.   ,, $B_1 = 70\cdot4°$ W.   ,,   ,, $8\cdot3°$

A comparison of these with the corresponding values given above shows that observation of disc B_2 from a relatively great distance has about the same effect as seeing it through a reduction screen.

Two factors determine the results of these last experiments. Just as the introduction of the black line in Hering's classical shadow experiment[1] modifies the impression, so in our experiments the colour-impression is changed when the observer is farther away. As a result of the greater distance, the *penumbrae* which contribute to the impression of *superimposed shadow* are no longer perceived in the same way as before. We may add the following observation to Hering's : The impression of shadow appears again within the black outline when the observer approaches the shadowed paper. The impression of shadow depends upon the size of the visual angle.[2] The change of size of the shadow is of greater significance in connection with the last experiments than is the change in the perception of the penumbra.

> Krauss has performed experiments upon the shadowing of surface colours in mescal intoxication ; it is an interesting fact that the shadow character is then repressed much more than it is in normal conditions.

The impression of shadowing[3] (and lighting) depends not only upon the conditions already discussed, but also,

---

[1] *Cf.* p. 50.   [2] *Cf.* § 46.

[3] For an extension of the foregoing experiments on shadowing *cf.* R. B. MacLeod, "An Experimental Investigation of Brightness Constancy," *Arch. of Psychol.*, 1932, 135.

in the following respects, upon the distribution of illumination in the visual field. If one particular illumination does not prevail throughout most of the visual field, we cannot have the impression of shadowing at the points of the visual field which are emitting less light. If the intensity of illumination is reduced throughout almost the entire visual field and only a small part is illuminated *normally*, we do not have the impression that the smaller part is normally illuminated and the rest of the field is in shadow. On the contrary, the total illumination of the visual field seems lower, whereas another spot of light seems superimposed at the normally illuminated point. The following observation may be made in this connection : With the shutters of the dark-room closed, open an Aubert diaphragm until you can perceive clearly the objects in the room. Now if daylight (not direct sunlight) falls through the diaphragm upon the floor of the dark-room, the observer has the impression that *light* is really lying upon the spot on the floor, while actually the spot is simply in normal illumination. If we open the window-shutter which holds the diaphragm, so that other parts of the floor are also lighted, the observer loses the impression that light is lying upon the floor, although the light-intensity is not reduced but somewhat increased, and sees the floor rather as normally illuminated. This observation shows that it depends upon the *distribution* of the " bright " and " dark " masses in the visual field whether an identically illuminated spot is apprehended as normally illuminated or is seen as covered by a spot of light. In his acute observations of lights lying upon coloured surfaces,[1] Hering has not gone into detail concerning the significance of the distribution of bright and dark masses in the visual field for the occurrence of these phenomena. We may describe here certain relevant observations which show, in part, a quite labile character.

Let us suppose that direct sunlight is falling upon a road, when the sun is high in the sky. The road and all the objects upon it then appear " too light " and, under

[1] Hering, VI, p. 9.

certain conditions, even blinding. Now let us assume
that the sun is behind us, so that we can see the " shadow "
cast by our body upon the road. The parts of the road
included in the shadow emit more light now than under
normal illumination, and seem, when we turn our attention
to them, to show us the " real " colour of the road ; but
when we observe the entire visual field, we have the
impression that there lies upon the shadowed parts a
darkness which does not really belong to the colour of the
road. Since most of the visual field appears in illumination
brighter than the normal and we are set for this total
brightness, colours which in themselves would be perceived
as normally illuminated now give the impression of
superimposed darkness. Now let us hold a large cardboard screen containing a small hole in such a position
that the shadow falls upon the road and the sunlight
passes through the opening. If we observe particular
parts of the shadow, we believe that we are apprehending
immediately the real colour of the road ; in the centre
of this real colour there is a spot of light which we can
easily perceive as standing out from the colour of the
ground. Our observations show that the apprehension
of colours as shadows or lights is, to a great extent,
independent of the absolute light-intensities of these
colours. As our first observation shows, when attention
is directed to the entire visual field, it depends upon what
illumination is considered to be prevalent.

One of Gelb's experiments, which he calls a " paradoxical " experiment,[1] is immediately and intimately
related to the present discussion. Gelb says in regard
to my shadowing experiments : " It is only when the
aperture-screen and the observer are in the same illumination as the black disc, which is displayed in full
daylight, that we can confirm these two observations,
viz., that the shadowed white disc is much whiter (under
direct observation) than the corresponding colour seen
through the aperture, and that the unshadowed black
disc retains approximately the quality of its colour as

[1] Gelb, p. 653 f.

seen through the aperture. . . . What, however, do we find when we reverse the conditions ? . . . Let us place the aperture-screen and the observer in an illumination which is reduced to that of the white disc. . . . Now what happens phenomenally when we turn from vision through the aperture to a free inspection of the discs ? The result is exactly the opposite of what was found before. After the aperture-screen is removed, the shadowed white disc appears in approximately the same quality (white) as the corresponding colour seen through the hole, while the unshadowed disc looks much too black. In this reversal-experiment we thus gain the impression that the subjective inequality was caused by a radical (subjective) modification on the normally illuminated side." Gelb explains that this reversal-experiment is no longer paradoxical if we abandon the assumption, which I had already postulated, that colour experiences in normal illumination do not present a problem in the same sense as do those appearing in non-normal illumination. I no longer adhere to this hypothesis, although at the same time we need not abandon the view that normal illumination and genuine colour occupy unique positions. Therefore I can agree entirely with Gelb's conclusions from the reversal-experiment that " we have no reason for ascribing to colour-vision in normal illumination any exceptional status in the genesis of our colour-perceptions " and that " colour-experiences in normal illumination are no more and no less ultimate and unexplainable than are those in non-normal illumination."

In the case of surface colours which are shadowed or lighted, it is easy to change the conditions of observation in such a way that the surface-character of the colours persists but they *no longer* appear as shadowed or lighted. We shall call this procedure *step-wise reduction*. For example, we may place an aperture-screen in such a position before a shadowed (or lighted) surface colour that we no longer observe any shadowing (or lighting), although we still perceive distinctly as a surface the colour appearing in the hole in the screen. The colour then appears at a definite distance from the eye, and may also have a non-frontal-parallel orientation to the observer. In general, the screen must be nearer to the coloured surface in this case than in reduction to film colour, in order that we may accommodate ourselves to the surface appearing in the hole. Under these conditions, we can no longer speak of a perception of a shadow (or light) extending over the surface ; the shadow (or the light) "fuses" entirely with the surface colour, giving the impression of a darker (or lighter) surface colour. According to my observations, this impression may be equated to that produced by a surface colour reflecting the same amount of light and standing in the same illumination as that of the reduction-screen. We reach this degree of darkness, for example, if we modify the shadow-impression as Hering did in his classical shadow-experiment. He produced step-wise reduction in his experiment not by the use of the aperture-screen but by the addition of a contour. This provides an occasion for me to remark that it makes no difference by what arrangement we bring about reduction, provided that the method of reduction is capable of bringing about a marked change in the colour-impression without changing the retinal excitation. In Hering's experiment, the shadowed spot becomes very dark because the paper seems to be "coloured grey with ink" and to have the same illumination as the rest of the paper. Step-wise reduction is thus connected here with reduction to the same illumination. If we use an aperture-screen for step-wise reduction of a shadowed paper, we do not always reach that darkening found in Hering's experiment. The paper usually appears somewhat brighter than its light-intensity would lead us to expect. The impression of shadow has, it is true, completely disappeared, but there remains the impression that the surface is illuminated *more weakly*. The fact that the paper appears somewhat brighter after step-wise reduction than after reduction to film colour is a simple consequence of this impression.

I

I shall report here some very significant results obtained by Gelb in his experiments on shadowing with his patient who had lost surface colours. Experiments on illumination perspective led to results of equal theoretical importance, so that I shall consider these too at this point. As regards colour-constancy, Gelb's patient behaved almost like a normal individual. The presence of clear-cut surface colours is thus unnecessary for constancy phenomena. The patient's behaviour was decidedly different from that of a normal individual, however, as regards superimposed lights and shadow-spots, neither of which he could apprehend as such. "For the patient the film colours of his environment were object colours, unless artificial experimental conditions made it impossible for him to refer the colours to objects as their bearers." "Without changing their spatial mode of appearance as such, the colours might or might not be referred by the patient to objects regarded as their bearers. When, for example, he looked through an aperture-screen, he saw only film colour without a bearer, but under normal conditions he saw a bearer appearing as a film colour. . . . Simply the consciousness that a colour is an object colour is sufficient for the appearance of phenomena of colour-constancy." "We have thus found that phenomena of colour-constancy may appear whenever object colours are seen. The particular spatial mode of appearance of the colours is, as such, without importance. The extent to which the colour-bearer appears organized seems, however, to be of striking significance for the appearance of some of the phenomena (spots of shadow and light) with which we are here concerned."[1] We recognize the importance of Gelb's discovery that the phenomena of colour-constancy can appear when the observer apprehends an object as a bearer of a colour and that the presence of a surface colour is not a *conditio sine qua non* for them. We should add, however, that the phenomena of colour-constancy are observable most distinctly and

[1] A. Gelb, "Über den Wegfall der Wahrnehmung von 'Oberflächenfarben'." *Zsch. f. Psychol.*, 1920, 84, p. 250.

most fully only when this consciousness of objectivity is founded on surface colours. That is shown, indeed, by the lack of certain phenomena in the case of Gelb's patient (absence of impressions of light and shadow). The experiment reported by Gelb himself[1] also seems to provide evidence of this.

§ 26. COLOUR-CONSTANCY AND PHOTOGRAPHY

W. Warstat has described certain differences between a picture of an object provided by a photographic plate and that which we get through vision.[2] From the point of view which we have adopted, many other points of difference are suggested. First of all, the photographic camera has no developing and maturing nervous substance. The human sense organ, with its nervous centres, represents an organism of the highest plastic power; its mechanical parallel, the photographic apparatus, " sees " objects for the thousandth time no differently from the first time. On account of this difference, it seemed instructive to me to undertake some " parallel experiments " with the human eye and the camera. If we wish to compare impressions given by the eye with pictures from the camera, we must naturally work with orthochromatic plates. We made two photographs of our experimental set-up described on p. 121. The first photograph (Fig. 7) of our apparatus was made after the two colours had been perfectly equated under reduction.[3] B_2 (the *left* colour-wheel in the photograph) was composed of $360°$ W. B_1 (the *right* colour-wheel in the photograph) had as setting I : $22°$ W, $338°$ B. In the photograph the grey colours on the two wheels are not different from each other; but the *observer* sees them as equally bright only *after* reduction. If we lift the reduction-screen and

---

[1] Cf., op. cit., p. 127.
[2] W. Warstat, *Allgemeine Aesthetik der photographischen Kunst auf psychologischer Grundlage.* Halle, 1909, pp. 9–28.
[3] In order that the disc might stand out more clearly from the background, we replaced the grey background used in the experiments by one considerably brighter.

look *directly* at colours which have been equated under reduction, we no longer see them as qualitatively equal, although the physical conditions are the same as those under which the photograph was made. We see B_2 as a strongly shadowed, almost white disc, and B_1 as an unshadowed, blackish grey or black disc. The photograph gives nothing of such an impression. If I look at the photograph without any further aids, the grey of the left disc appears no different from that of the right disc. We do, however, perceive clearly a shadowing of the part of the apparatus lying to the left of the shadow-casting screen, although this shadow appears to be completely *fused* with the colours upon which it is lying. If we attend not to the quality but to the insistence of the colours of the disc in setting I (Fig. 7), we may find that it is equally great on the two sides. Since there is a similar equality between the colours of the discs in the photograph, we may say that photography reproduces *correctly* the relationships of achromatic colours in *insistence.*

The second photograph (Fig. 8) of the set-up was made after the two discs had been set for the *same quality* by an observer looking at them *directly*, as in the experiments described above.[1] The values of setting II were : $B_1 = 120° W$, $240° B$. In the light of our explanation of the first photograph, this second one will immediately be clear. The picture reproduces the relationships of the two discs in insistence ; and if I judge the two discs, which are adjusted for the same quality, in terms of the extent to which I feel myself affected by each, there is a significant difference resembling that in the photograph. In the latter case, we cannot, of course, speak in any sense of qualitative identity, the one surface being light grey and the other dark grey. We may conclude from this photograph, as from the first, that photography can never provide impressions of achromatic colours differing in pronouncedness.

Photography provides only a unidimensional series of

[1] *Cf.* p. 123 ff.

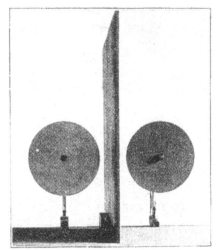

Fig. 7

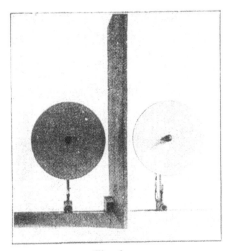

Fig. 8

[face p. 132

achromatic colours, whereas these colours appear in various degrees of pronouncedness when we are looking at the things themselves. The reason is this : photography cannot utilize certain determinants which have measurable influence upon the character of normal perception, or at least cannot utilize them to the same extent. The photographer must take account of this fact, since it is not determined by any accidental peculiarity of *our* photographs but lies in the very nature of photography itself.

Let us consider now some of the reasons why photographs can never give perfectly natural impressions.[1]

1. Photography presents a " sector " of the world, and can reproduce relationships of colour and of illumination only within this sector. Aside from certain exceptional cases, it rules out all those determinants of colour-perception which originate in the *total constellation*, e.g., in the position of the observer in relation to the objects he is seeing. In normal perception of colour and illumination this position is always of influence. Since we know, for example, that under normal conditions light enters a room through the window, we should be not a little surprised, in looking at our apparatus, to find the disc standing near the window shaded and the other unshaded. Such determinants of the perception of colours and of their illumination are lacking *a priori* in photography. It is true that there is a certain regularity in the distribution of light and shade and a certain logic of illumination in a photograph, but this regularity holds only within the frame of the picture. It is of interest that a contradiction in the light-distribution in the visual field (such as we just assumed to be possible for the natural appearance of things) [2] does not appear between the type of distribution of light in the photograph and that in its neighbourhood. Let us suppose that we have a picture in

---

[1] In this connection we are disregarding entirely the lack of hues and are considering only achromatic colours.

[2] Sometimes I have observed contradictory light-distribution in the visual field when I have looked into an invisible mirror and seen mirrored objects in conditions of illumination different from those existing for the objects in the neighbourhood of the mirror. Here we may also mention the impression of illumination which we get when an intaglio appears as a cameo. " That produces a kind of *supernatural illumination* [italics mine] of the relief which seems, as it were, to arise from its interior." Helmholtz, II, p. 772.

which the observer sees the light falling from *left to right*; the picture does not lose its effect in the least if we hang it in a room in which the light is falling from *right to left*. We cannot speak of a contradiction of illumination such as we should experience in perceiving the situation postulated above. These points are perhaps sufficient to demonstrate that determinants which are important in the apprehension of colour-relationships in the real world cease to be effective in the photographic sector. The question which we have discussed here recurs in exactly the same form as regards the fidelity to nature of a *painting*.

2. Photographs of objects are ordinarily much smaller than the objects themselves, so that they appear in photographs under visual angles which are too small and hence unusual. One consequence of this is that the various parts of an object appear in a photograph in degrees of distinctness different from those present in the perception of the objects themselves. This fact is not without significance for the kinds of colour which appear in objects. I have performed experiments to determine to what extent colours and *distribution of light* may appear more natural when a photograph is observed through a system of lenses which causes the objects to appear in life-size. When I looked at photographs through such an apparatus, I noted that all the attributes of the colours and illumination came to resemble reality more closely.

3. Even with *binocular* vision, spatial relationships within the photographic sector appear similar to those in normal *monocular* vision (if the eye is stationary). Binocular vision may lead either directly or indirectly (through a more distinct perception of depth) to higher colour-constancy. In any case, the lack of retinal disparity in perception of photographs explains in part why the colours of photographs or objects differ from those of the objects themselves. We are able to confirm our hypothesis in two ways. (*a*) Monocular instead of binocular perception of a situation should cause colour-constancy to recede and colour-impressions to become similar to those presented in photographs. This assumption will be confirmed by experiments.[1] (*b*) A stereoscopic picture seen in a stereoscope should be more " real " in its colouring than a non-stereoscopic picture made under otherwise similar conditions. Experience confirms this supposition. When we look at photographs in the stereo-

[1] *Cf.* § 34.

scope, the light-distribution stands out more clearly; also the shadows become more diffuse and are severed to a greater degree from the colours of the objects.

§ 27. INDIVIDUAL DIFFERENCES

We had the opportunity, in lecture-demonstrations, to perform a group-experiment on the shadowing of achromatic surface colours. For B_2 I selected a white disc and a strong shadow. Then I set Value I to satisfy myself. The participants in the demonstration saw this setting first, and all accepted the equation which I had made. Then, while the observers remained in the same position, I lifted the reduction screen and permitted them to survey the conditions of illumination. Also I mentioned that the settings on the colour-wheels themselves had not been changed. Then all the observers without exception agreed that the shadowed colour was now distinctly brighter than the unshadowed colour, although the brightening of the shadowed colours appeared in quite different degrees for the various observers. While some were content with mentioning a rather distinct brightening, others could not express adequately their surprise concerning the brightening of the shadowed colour and wished to be shown repeatedly this " remarkable phenomenon." This demonstration should show that in experiments of this sort we must, as a rule, allow for great individual differences.[1] We shall discuss these in greater detail below.

What is to be said about individual differences in our shadowing experiment? Let us take, for example, the first experiment with each of the two observers, R and U. In these two experiments, the brightness of the shaded disc B_2 was exactly the same, and the intensity of its shadowing approximately the same, as Values I show. We obtained 11·8 and 7·1 as the retinal values

---

[1] For a detailed study of individual differences in connection with various constancy phenomena, cf. R. H. Thouless, " Individual Differences in Phenomenal Regression," Brit. J. Psychol., 1932, 22.

of central brightening for R and U respectively. This difference is surprisingly high.

We come now to individual differences in the experiments on illumination perspective and the experiments with the episcotister. The settings of the reduced values are accepted by all observers; therefore, if we start with the same reduction-values, the individual differences should be expressed in the quotients of the brightness series, as well as in those of the retinal series. We shall limit ourselves to a comparison of the values obtained from the four observers in those cases in which the same settings were used on disc A.

	Observer		Brightness Values			
			M	L	K	N
1.	Disc A :	360° W .	0·36	0·49	0·62	0·88
2.	„	270° W .	0·35	0·49	0·60	0·87
3.	„	210° W .	0·31	0·49	0·64	0·80
4.	„	180° W .	0·30	0·48	0·54	0·77
5.	„	100° W .	0·27	0·38	0·45	0·60
6.	„	80° W .	0·25	0·33	0·40	0·62
7.	„	60° W .	0·27	0·30	0·41	0·65

We have arranged the four series in such a way that the one with the lowest values stands first and that with the highest values last. The differences expressed between the series of M and N are enormous. The values of L and K fall between these extremes. Thus great individual differences appear in experiments on illumination perspective, as well as in the experiments on shadowing.

We shall give, finally, the series of values obtained in the experiments with the episcotister.

Observers	Brightness Series		Retinal Series	
	P	$M\ddot{u}$	P	$M\ddot{u}$
E 90° .	0·336	0·388	1·34	1·55
E 30° .	0·284	0·298	3·41	3·58
E 10° .	0·243	0·306	9·16	11·02
E 3° .	0·238	0·189	28·60	23·70

Since the surface colours to be compared stood under exactly the same conditions of illumination for the two observers, the brightness and retinal series should express the individual differences in the same way.[1] This was actually the case. With episcotister openings of from 90° to 10° the individual differences are in a direction opposite that for the opening 3°. The individual differences are greater for openings of 3° and 10° than for those of 30° and 90°. Since the relative brightening is always higher with a small opening of the episcotister than with a large opening, we may suspect that *individual differences are greatest when colour-constancy reaches its highest values.*

All authors who have performed experiments on colour-constancy have been able to confirm the fact that individual differences are extraordinarily high in comparison with those in other visual experiments, but the hypothesis which I have just expressed has met with no agreement. Brunswik has dealt in detail with such individual differences.[2] He claims to have found that individual differences were smallest in those groups of observers who showed the highest degrees of colour-constancy and were greatest when colour-constancy was of moderate value. In the experiments performed by Burzlaff, neither my hypothesis nor Brunswik's could be confirmed.

We have introduced the method of reduction in order to compare with each other the retinal processes corresponding to colour impressions of various kinds. If two colours appear the same after reduction to the same illumination, their difference *before* reduction must be due to a difference between the central factors corresponding to them. We have shown that equations made under reduction are generally accepted. Since this is not true of equations made before reduction, it follows that the change undergone centrally by the neural excitations emanating from the retina is of different kinds or magnitudes for the different observers.

We assume that the mode of functioning of the peripheral mechanisms of the visual organ remains

[1] *Cf.* p. 136.   [2] *Zsch. f. Psychol.*, 1928, 109.

essentially unchanged after birth. This does not hold, however, for those conditions in the nervous sector which may intrench upon the psychophysical processes underlying colour-perception. Among these factors we may include the physiological processes underlying perception of form and space, as well as processes of other types, such as those determined by memory colours (§ 32).. If such modes of apprehension become habitual, they may lead to more or less fixed attitudes which profoundly influence colour-perception. Let us pick out a few of the well-defined modes of apprehending colours. The psychologist who is studying colour has obviously quite a different attitude toward colour from that of the layman, and the painter in turn, with his deeply rooted interest in colours, sees the world with eyes different from those of the psychologist. Owing to the variety of possible attitudes toward colour, it is not difficult to arrive at a satisfying explanation of the individual differences which may be found. Since types of apprehension, whether they be fleeting or lasting, differ from person to person, we obtain differing values in experiments such as those we have described. It may be enlightening to illustrate these general principles in the concrete case of the painter's vision. If we assume that it is the business of the painter to reproduce the world in its natural constitution, it follows that he must be expert in seeing colours as they should be painted upon the canvas. He must endeavour to see the world as a picture. That leads him, even without any particular reductive mechanisms, to apprehend colours in their reduced values. He must refer colours (in reduced form) to a fictitious surface with fictitious illumination. The painter's attitude is directed as far as possible toward the perception of " colour as such " and as little as possible toward perception of " objects." That is clear to anyone who has become at all interested in the problems of colour-production by the painter. We can support what we have just said by referring to the observations of Fuchs. One of his observers, Professor Cornelius, differed in all his reports from the others and, as we may express it briefly, in the direction of reduced vision. Now Professor Cornelius is a painter, and it is from this fact that Fuchs explains the discrepancy. " It is at once clear that in painters, who must represent objective space in one plane, a type of vision must be developed which differs from that of naïve observation. It is possible that due to an habitual attitude they see natural colours as relatively filmy." [1] As for our own observers, no one was set for " colour as such " and no one for pure object perception ; yet even though these extremes were lacking, there was sufficient range for individual dispersion.

Gelb has also expressed himself with reference to the problem of individual differences. " Under these different experimental conditions, we have in the last analysis differences in the richness and specific character of the organization and articulation of visual space. An explanation of the great individual differences is also to be sought in the same direction. . . . This explanation does not lie in the differences between the various observers due to past experience, but in the change and lability of inner attitudes and the correspondingly different configurations of the visual field." [2]

These individual differences in vision can appear only when we are dealing with a comparison of colours standing under *different* conditions of illumination. If this is not the case, and the colours are standing under the same conditions of illumination, even though these may not be normal, we cannot expect that the attitudes which the various observers assume in equating colours will differ significantly from each other in any respect. In these experiments we are to a certain extent, of course, in a subjective realm. Even if two impressions are largely subject to the influence of modes of reaction differing from one individual to another, the *two* excitations emanating from the retina will undergo the same influence whenever the same central factors are effective in the two cases. It is possible to study these individual

[1] Fuchs, I, p. 225. [2] Gelb, p 677.

differences experimentally only if the factors determining them are in such a way operative as to have *objective significance*.

It is hardly possible to determine experimentally to what extent individual differences appear in connection with the distinctness of other modes of appearance of colour (lustre, volume colour, transparency, etc.). Such differences might very well exist for those modes of appearance which are influenced by configural factors.

§ 28. COLOUR-CONSTANCY AND THE CONCEPT OF ILLUSION

If we did not realize that the colour-phenomena which we have treated are governed by definite laws, we might tend to consider them as no more than curiosities of perception. By some writers (*e.g.*, Sully) they are simply considered illusions. ". . . when I look at a sheet of white paper in a feebly-lit room, I seem to see its whiteness. If, however, I bring it near the window, and let the sun fall on a part of it, I at once recognize that what I have been seeing is not white, but a decided grey."[1] I shall disregard the fact that Sully must have made a false observation in this case, in so far as the effect observable in experiments is quite opposed to his description ; I should simply like to mention, in connection with this observation that we should be using the concept of illusion too broadly and without sufficient justification if, following Sully, we were to call all changes of colour appearing under change of illumination illusions of perception. According to Sully's view, almost all of the results we have given would have to be attributed to perceptual illusions. To be consistent, we should have to say that an observer who calls a strongly shadowed white surface " white " is subject to the strongest illusion. It seems to me, however, that that would be reversing the actual state of affairs. I am subject to an illusion only when I apprehend a situation

[1] J. Sully, *Illusions*, London, 4th ed., 1894, p. 88.

falsely, yet here the observer who calls the colour " white " is certainly closest to a knowledge of the true state of affairs. Those organic mechanisms by which our experiences are formed in greatest possible independence of peripheral stimuli obviously serve to prevent illusions. It is not difficult to discover motives which might lead us to speak of perceptual illusions in the cases we have described ; we may be thinking in these cases of the *intensities of the retinal images*. We are, of course, subject to great error if we ascribe to the retinal image of a shadowed white disc the same light intensity as to a qualitatively identical but normally illuminated surface. The intensity of a retinal image, however, usually evades observation and can be compared with that of another only after reduction. Even if we were to make the relationships after reduction a measure of how the observer has judged, we should be neglecting the fact that retinal excitations never appear in isolation but always within a total field ; as we shall demonstrate later (§ 65), one and the same retinal excitation may lead to different colour-impressions, depending upon the total excitation of the retina. Real illusions—such as misreading—are marked by their lability ; they disappear under a high degree of attention. Such lability is not, in general, to be found in our phenomena. It is proper to speak of an illusion of perception if the *memory colour*[1] of an object has such striking influence upon colour-vision that we are led into an error regarding the bearer of this colour ; but it is characteristic even in this case that the perceived colour may be *completely changed* by a change of attention.

§ 29. COLOUR-CONSTANCY AND EXPOSITION TIME

If, using a tachistoscope, I look at an object in normal illumination, sometimes for a longer and sometimes for a shorter time, I am unable to recognize any distinct influence of the length of the time upon the colour.

[1] *Cf.* § 32.

Surface colours lying in a visual field which is partially in *non-normal* illumination behave differently. Even superficial inspection shows that their appearance changes as the exposition time is varied. *Within certain limits, a shortening of the exposition time causes colour-constancy to recede.*

The apparatus used in § 25 was supplemented by a tachistoscopic mechanism. In front of the reduction-screen, which always remained lifted in these tachistoscopic experiments, was a double fall-screen. This device consisted of two cardboard screens, held up by means of electromagnets, which at first covered the object to be exposed. When the electrical circuit supplying one electromagnet was opened and the first screen fell, the object was exposed and remained visible until the circuit of the other electromagnet was opened and the second screen fell. We used four exposition times—$t_1 = 0.6$; $t_2 = 1.1$; $t_3 = 1.7$; and $t_4 = 3.4$ sec. The shadow, which remained the same throughout the experiment, corresponded to that of the A-experiments.[1] The procedure was the same as that in the experiments on shadowing. We shall also use similar symbols.

	Value	I	Disc	$B_1 = 27.6°$ W
Exposition Time t_1	,,	II	,,	$B_1 = 38.5°$ W
,, ,, t_2	,,	II	,,	$B_1 = 56.4°$ W
,, ,, t_3	,,	II	,,	$B_1 = 61.4°$ W
,, ,, t_4	,,	II	,,	$B_1 = 77.4°$ W

One might raise the objection that the differences among Values II are brought about not by changes undergone by the *shadowed* disc through variation of the exposition time but by changes in the *normally illuminated disc*. The only changes undergone by surface colours in a normally illuminated visual field which might be significant here would be those resulting from the rise of the excitation. The rise of the excitation is completed, however, in periods of time less than the shortest exposition times employed here. We can also convince ourselves immed-

---

[1] *Cf.* p. 123 ff.

iately that we may reduce the exposition time even below t_1 without noticing any change in the colour of B_1, while such experiments with B_2 give quite different results. Thus we may consider our results to be an expression of modifications undergone by disc B_2 as the exposition time is varied.

The conditions of observation in t_4 are most related to those of the earlier A-experiments (observers R and U), in which the exposition time was about 3 sec. Within such periods, the observer is able to make a comparative judgment of the two discs without haste. In these cases we shall form, as before, the brightness quotients B and Q ; they are 0·23 and 0·25 respectively. These quotients are significantly lower than the corresponding values of the earlier observers ; this might be traced primarily to the weaker shadowing of B_2.[1] The B and Q values for the results obtained with the various exposition times are as follows :

		t_4	t_3	t_2	t_1
B Values	.	0·23	0·19	0·17	0·12
Q Values	.	2·5	2·0	1·9	1·3

Arranged in this order, the B and Q series manifest distinctly decreasing values, *i.e.*, *with decreasing exposition time, colour - constancy is reduced.* Repetition of the experiments with other observers confirmed this conclusion.

In so far as colour-constancy is lowered when exposition time is shortened, we may also consider *the shortening of exposition time to be a reductive procedure.*

The Values II formed decreasing series of values from t_4 to t_1. What values do we get if we shorten the exposition time still more ? It is probable *a priori* that with further shortening of the time we should at a certain point reach a limit beyond which the impression of the shadowed disc would no longer change. The brightness of the shadowed disc cannot be less than the brightness of the impression brought about by an equally intense stimulus

[1] *Cf.* Values I.

with an equally short exposition time in a normally
illuminated visual field. It is, however, questionable
whether this limit is really reached. In the following
experiments, we used very short exposition times. Since
it is impossible in such short times to look from one disc
to the other, we had to resort to a successive presentation
of the two discs.

At some distance from B_2 stood a photographic shutter
with an opening of such breadth that when the observer
was quite near it he could conveniently look through with
both eyes at the shadowed disc. The observer always
looked first at the shadowed disc and then at the normally
illuminated disc, the exposition time for the latter *not*
being limited. The exposition times were varied by
changing the tension of the spring and the height of the
opening of the instantaneous shutter. We were able in
this way to get times varying from 0·05 to 0·0005 sec.
After I had begun the experiments in the way I have
described, it proved to be very difficult to set upon the
variable disc by the method of limits a colour which was
equal to the colour of the disc exposed briefly. I was
more successful in attaining this end by another procedure.
After exposing the shadowed disc, I presented in normal
illumination the above-described[1] scale of achromatic
colours and had the observer match the colour observed
on the shadowed disc with a member of the scale or place
it between two members of the scale.

With the shortest exposition time—about 0·0005 sec.—
the shadowed disc was not perceived at all. Even with
the next longer time—0·0017 sec.—it could not always
be seen. This is due, in part, to the fact that no fixation
point could be established and ocular movements could
not be made in these short periods of time. It is more
probable, however, that it was the weakness of the light
emitted by the shadowed disc and its weak contrast with
the background which made the disc imperceptible.
When objects are bright and stand out in sufficiently
strong contrast to the background, they are always

[1] *Cf.* p. 77.

perceptible, even with an exposition time as short as 0·0005 sec. Even without a fixation point, the observers soon became able to perceive the shadowed disc in almost every exposure when the exposition time was at least 0·0036 sec.

Four observers took part in the experiments. When the shadowed disc was seen at all in the experiments with an exposition time of 0·0017, the observers' selections of equivalents from the scale of eighteen colours[1] varied between the following steps :

Observer K: 9–12 ; Ma: 8–11 ; B: 7–8 ; E: 9–11.

I had so regulated the intensity of illumination of the shadowed disc that after reduction it appeared approximately equal to a normally illuminated velvet-black (with a brightness value of $6°\ W$). For this reason, the values obtained from the various observers may easily be compared with each other. Since our problem is to find the lowest limit to which colour-constancy may fall when the exposition time is very short, we shall select simply the lowest value found for each of the observers. In terms of the brightness values of the papers of the scale, we obtained the following B and Q values :

	K	B	Ma	E
B Values	0·27	0·14	0·18	0·27
Q Values	15·9	8·4	10·7	15·9

The result is somewhat astonishing. *Even with an exposition time so short that the shadowed disc is barely perceptible, colour-constancy persists to a considerable degree.* As for the results with the other exposition times (1/20, 1/48, 1/110, and 1/160 sec.), we may say that a variation of the exposition time within these limits was without any determinable influence for observer K, but that for the other observers there was undeniably a slight

---

[1] I have denoted the members of the scale by the numbers from 1 to 18 ; their values in terms of the colour-wheel are rounded off to integral degrees : (1) 6° ; (2) 10° ; (3) 15° ; (4) 25° ; (5) 34° ; (6) 41° ; (7) 51° ; (8) 64° ; (9) 80° ; (10) 96° ; (11) 114° ; (12) 154° ; (13) 185° ; (14) 219° ; (15) 259° ; (16) 289° ; (17) 327° ; (18) 360° W.

brightening of the shadowed disc as the time became greater. Since our method was not suited to the determination of exact values, we have refrained from giving particular numbers. We were unable to follow up the course of the results for times between 0·05 and 0·6 sec., but there is no apparent reason why there should be any irregularity in this intermediate region. We may conclude from our experiments that colour-constancy is reduced as the exposition time is shortened to a point at which the shadowed disc is still barely perceptible. This conclusion is apparently contradicted by the results of observer K, the only observer from whom we obtained results with an exposition time of 0·6 sec. and with the shortest time which we used. While the value of Q was 15 for the shortest exposition time, it amounted to only 3 for $t = 0·6$ sec. We should remark in connection with this contradiction that the various intensities of illumination of the shadowed surface colours do not permit immediate comparison. Under otherwise similar conditions, as we have shown, Q becomes greater as the shadow becomes deeper. We have a measure for the latter in the reduced values of the shadowed discs. In the experiments with $t = 0·6$ sec., the reduced value was $15·6° W$; with $t = 0·0017$ sec., $6° W$. This difference alone would thus tend to make Q considerably greater when the exposition time is rather short. There is in these experiments, however, still another factor working in the same direction. The experiments result quite differently depending upon whether we present only *one* colour for comparison (as in the method of limits) or present at the same time a whole scale of colours (as in the experiments with short t). Under the latter conditions, the observer selects a much brighter colour to match the shadowed colour. In connection with this point we shall report particular experiments. The above-mentioned contradiction is shown to be only apparent if we take these two facts into consideration.

How can we explain this decrease of colour-constancy resulting from a shortening of the exposition time?

First of all, I believe that I can show that this decrease is essentially bound up with a difference of illumination in the visual field—in particular, with a difference which causes a normal illumination to dominate, while a weaker illumination is presented only in a smaller part of the field. The phenomena are decidedly different when we shorten the exposition time of a visual field which is uniformly illuminated throughout. I shall report the following experiment concerning this point. If I look from a room through an instantaneous shutter upon a street which is normally illuminated in its entire extent, or is lighted directly by sunlight, then even with the shortest time of 0·0005 sec., the objects are seen in approximately their usual colour and in that illumination which is also perceived with longer exposition times. This is true even if the illumination is weaker than the normal (provided it is not too much weaker). The experiment shows also how quickly the impression of a particular illumination of the visual field may appear. In the present connection, it is particularly interesting that neither the colouring nor the impression of illumination is changed in any way worthy of mention when the exposition time is very much reduced, provided that the illumination in the entire visual field is unitary. Let us pass from this to a second fact, which is important for the explanation of our results. The sector of the street which is seen through the shutter is changed in such a way that it loses in reality-character and assumes rather the character of a picture. What causes this change ? The *depth-impression* of the situation is changed, somewhat as it is when we pass from binocular to monocular vision.[1] Space appears decidedly shallower and a particular object no longer so plastic. The contours of objects are no longer given in their original sharpness. Those configural characteristics which support the impression of materiality can no longer be apprehended with assurance, so that all the objects are, as in a picture,

---

[1] *Cf.* the analogous observations of L. v. Karpinska, *Zsch. f. Psychol.*, 1910, 57.

stripped extensively of their materiality. The mode of appearance of the colours approaches that of film colour. All in all, reality seems degraded into an impressionistic picture.[1] What will be the influence of such a reorganization of the visual field under shortening of the exposition time if illumination is not unitary but is such as we used in our experiments ? Obviously a shortening of the exposition time must change the colours of the abnormally illuminated parts of the field as if they were reduced to the prevailing illumination. The shorter the exposition time is, the more this levelling of illumination must take effect. We thus find in our quantitative experiments what we should expect in the light of these considerations ; we have, therefore, an explanation for our results.[2]

The shortest exposition times force the observer to accept passively what the visual field offers ; a free exposition time permits him to " work over " the visual field. When presented with a shadowed disc, for example, he has an active feeling of " remoulding." When no time limit is set, this activity obviously contributes not a little to the heightening of the reality-character of our experiences.

This active attitude toward a visual impression always means an attempt to reorganize the visual field. Not all visual fields lend themselves equally to that activity. A normally illuminated surface, whose microstructure may be seen quite distinctly, is not a very suitable object for subjective revision. The more unusual the illumination is, the more adaptable are the objects seen in it ; this is shown with particular distinctness in chromatic illumination. In all cases of colour perception involving this " activity " of the observer, the resulting reorganiza-

---

[1] Experimental studies of the impressionistic type of vision may be linked with these observations under very short exposition times. *Cf.* E. R. Jaensch, *Zsch. f. Sinnesphysiol.*, 1923, 54.

[2] " Every means of unifying the impression of illumination must have an effect similar to that of the aperture-screen, even if this unification does not concern the objective illuminations, but only the impression of illumination. This explains why, under certain conditions, we may, even without a reduction-screen, see a white paper in relatively weak illumination and a . . . black paper in relatively strong illumination more or less as they would appear in a photometer." Gelb, p. 676.

tions of the visual field are the real causes for the observed changes in colour-constancy.

Experiments with tachistoscopic exposition of colours of other modes of appearance were not carried out systematically, but only incidentally. With very short exposition times, volume colours become less voluminous and more filmy. The transparence of colours becomes less distinct, the transparent colours fusing with the colours seen through them. Lustrous lights " adhere " more and more to the lustrous objects, and at the same time appear more luminous. These changes are not surprising, since we have already come to know the change in the mode of appearance of surface colours with very short exposition times. Even with the very shortest exposition times, film colours do not change their mode of appearance, although their localization becomes still more indefinite. Luminous colours also retain their character even with very short exposition times. These facts concerning the various degrees of destructive effect resulting from tachistoscopic exposition are of some significance for an understanding of the genesis of these colour phenomena.

§ 30. REMARKS ON METHODOLOGY

We proposed above[1] to perform experiments to determine what influence there may be when, with short exposition time, the disc B_1 is not compared with single colours by the method of limits, but is seen simultaneously with an entire scale of achromatic colours. I shall report the results of the experiments carried out with observer B.

$B_2 = 360° W$. Deep shadow.

I. Determination by the method of limits. $n = 4$. $B_1 = 151\cdot4° W$
II. Determination by the scale method. $n = 4$. $B_1 = 289\cdot7° W$[2]

---

[1] *Cf.* p. 146.
[2] These values are mean values of the brightnesses of four members of the scale which the observer matched in turn with B_2. I have retained the symbol B_1.

$B_2 = 180° W$.   Deep shadow.

  I. Determination by the method of limits. $n = 4$. $B_1 = 43.4° W$
 II. Determination by the scale method. $n = 4$. $B_1 = 59.5° W$

The differences between the brightness-values obtained by the two methods are $289.7° W - 151.4° W = 138.3° W$, and $59.5° W - 43.4° W = 16.1° W$. Particularly the first difference, which interests us in connection with the experiments described above, is extraordinarily large. This value might furnish the solution of the contradiction mentioned above.[1]

Experiments with the scale method led me to give Burzlaff the problem of following up certain questions of methodology. I shall give here, as I have already promised, a résumé of some of his main results.

Burzlaff used the apparatus for illumination perspective under daylight illumination. The illumination was reduced to about 1/20. Taking these general conditions as his basis, Burzlaff distinguishes four constellations, which he calls A, B, C and D. In constellation A, as in my experiments on illumination perspective, two variable discs were used. The spatial arrangement of the discs in constellation B was the opposite of that in C; otherwise B and C were alike. Both B and C differed from A in the following respect: a variable disc was used for one colour-impression, but the other was replaced by a chart of forty-eight achromatic colours arranged according to brightness. It was the same chart which had already been used in the observations described in § 14. The experimental situation D was distinguished from B and C in that the disc which had been retained in B and C was now replaced by a second chart of colours. On this second chart, however, the forty-eight small squares of colour were placed in random arrangement, yet in such a way that they formed twelve lines of four colours each. The process of comparison in constellation A was the method of limits, as also used in my experiments. " If charts replace discs, the procedure is as follows : the

---

[1] *Cf.* p. 146 f.

colour on the unarranged chart which is used as the principal colour is marked by a drawing-pencil. Using a wooden pointer, the experimenter runs through the other series, in which the greys are arranged according to brightness. . . . The pointer is moved so slowly that the observer has sufficient time to make comparisons. . . ." In B and C, matches were made between the colour set up on the disc and a colour of the chart, and in D between colours of the two charts. Both adults and children observed in these experiments.

The results from the adults in constellation A agree essentially with those which I obtained by the same method.[1] All the brightness-quotients remained distinctly below 1, $i.e.$, there was in no case an ideal colour-constancy. The results confirmed our generalization that white and its neighbours are the colours which retain their character most stably in weak illumination. In constellation B there was a marked rise in the brightness-quotients. " There appears, indeed, the surprising result that the brightness-quotients of all the observers are on the average larger than 1, if we disregard the colours at the black and white ends of the grey scale. A member of the black-white series standing under greatly reduced illumination appears brighter than a normally illuminated member of the black-white series of the same white valence. Colour-constancy is ideal ($i.e.$, 1) for the brightest member (360°) ; as the white component decreases, the brightness-quotient rises above 1 to 1·38 in the case of 183° and then, toward the black end, falls a few hundredths of a unit below 1. . . . It is striking that in this constellation the more weakly illuminated colours appear, in general, as brighter than those standing in normal illumination. Such a result has hitherto never been found." In constellation C (involving a reversal of the spatial arrangement of B), " the brightness-quotient falls as we pass from white to black, from 1 to 0·51, $i.e.$, in almost ideal proportion to the white valences of th colours." " What Katz calls ideal colour-constancy is

[1] $Cf.$ § 19.

found in situation D. The brightness-quotients lie not more than a few hundredths of a unit below or above 1. . . . The values seem to give evidence that here we have, in certain respects, the type of colour-perception which is most closely related to that of everyday life." In summary, Burzlaff finds that " there is a high dependence of the degree of colour-constancy upon the method of investigation, in so far as the latter is an occasion for the creation of different configurations of the visual field and configurations which are effective under different conditions."

" The results for the adults and for the children agree well in constellations B, C and D. Only the results in situation A (not in B, C or D) would lead us to conclude that there is a development of colour-constancy in the course of individual life." We are disregarding, for the time being, the question of the development of colour-constancy ; we shall return to the question below.

Now how does Burzlaff explain these differences between the different constellations ? He begins with the asumption that D is the constellation most related to life. " That is justified, because in this case the two visual fields . . . manifest the highest degree of articulation. Katz has often emphasized how significant it is for the highest possible degree of colour-constancy that the visual field be filled with numerous objects easily distinguishable from each other. . . . The more homogeneously the visual field is filled, the more the phenomena of colour-constancy recede. . . ." Burzlaff points out quite rightly that the great richness of articulation in the two charts, the normally and the weakly illuminated, would lead us to expect *a priori* an approximately ideal matching of the corresponding members. The results in the other constellations are to be understood in terms of this case. ' Let us return first to constellation A. " In the two fields to be compared in A, there is, as contrasted with D, an extensive impoverishment of articulation. That must have as a result the reduction of colour-constancy. . . . Will the reduction not act in the same direction in the two fields . . . ? That would be expected only if the two visual fields had the same intensity of illumination. That is not, however, the case, one field being more strongly illuminated than the other. We should bear in mind that with approximately the same articulation, the field standing under weaker illumination must undergo relatively greater change as colour-constancy recedes; then, if the two fields are combined into one (they adjoin each other and consequently the nearer one will appear brighter and the farther darker), the farther (or more weakly illuminated) field must become darker. This corresponds to our expectation, based upon such theoretical considerations, that all brightness-quotients should be smaller in A than in D." Burzlaff then discusses the differences between C and D. All quotients, up to a value of 360°, are lower in C than in D. That becomes intelligible if we compare the constellations not directly but indirectly in terms of constellation A. A and C differ in that in the one case a colour-wheel and in the other a chart is standing under the weaker illumination. "In both cases, however, a colour-wheel is presented under normal illumination. We may assume, therefore, that this factor exercises the same influence in the two cases. We should thus obtain differences similar to those between A and C if we simply set the wheel and chart next to each other under the inferior conditions of illumination and compared the brightnesses of the two coloured objects." When Burzlaff carried out experiments to answer this question, he found his hypothesis confirmed. "We discovered the interesting fact that there is a darkening tendency when achromatic colours are seen simultaneously side by side under weak illumination; this darkening tendency appears most strongly in the middle grey steps." Burzlaff now applies this result and discovers that particularly the results in C, which deviate very considerably from ideal colour-constancy, appear intelligible. "The darkening influence of the comparison chart of forty-eight colours in C depresses the total brightness-level of the field standing in reduced illumination and thereby causes the normally illuminated field to appear relatively brighter, *i.e.*, the brightness-quotients must fall. If our assumption is correct, then in *B* (which involves a reversal of the spatial arrangement of *C*) the darkening tendency of the brightness-articulation of the chart must have an opposite effect . . . and in *D*, in which the darkening tendencies effective in *B* and *C* are acting antagonistically, their effects must be approximately equalized. As a matter of fact, the brightness-quotient in *D* occupy an intermediate position; they are significantly greater in *B* and considerably lower in *C*." For details of the explanation the reader must consult the original work.

§ 31. Colour-Constancy and Visual Configuration

More than other authors, Burzlaff has demonstrated the unusually complicated interrelation of two factors which together determine the results of experiments on colour-constancy—articulation of the visual field, and method of comparison. In what follows, I shall discuss certain studies which have dealt with the significance of configuration of the visual field for colour-constancy; the writers do not always realize that the method of comparison changes as configuration changes. Cramer found that the introduction of a figure into the visual field leads to higher colour-constancy. "Through the introduction of the disc, the subjective brightness—and hence the transformation—becomes considerably greater." [1] Granit has referred to the significance of the presence of a figure for the impression of illumination. "It is of great significance for the formation of the impression of illumination that a figure be seen in the illuminated region." [2] One of Katona's studies [3] represents a noteworthy contribution to our problem. Into a small,

[1] T. Cramer, *Zsch. f. Sinnesphysiol.*, 1922, 54.
[2] R. Granit, *op. cit.*
[3] *Psychol. Forsch.*, 1929, 12.

abnormally illuminated visual field he brought, in succession, six different objects and tested the effect of each upon colour-constancy. He used the following objects : (*a*) a photograph ; (*b*) two green postage-stamps ; (*c*) a hatched surface with writing on it ; (*d*) the negative of the photograph ; (*e*) a picture of a trunk ; and (*f*) a picture of a house standing upside down. Katona distinguishes three groups of factors which support colour-constancy :

1. Figural articulation or form-configuration.
   (*a*) Mutual demarcation, clear contours.
   (*b*) Object-character, figure as opposed to ground.

2. Colour-configuration.[1]
   (*a*) Surface colours.
   (*b*) Mutual demarcation of colours, pronouncedness of colour attributes.

3. Familiarity of the object.

In the light of what we shall have to say in the next section about memory colours, it is noteworthy that although Katona does not hold that figural factors must be familiar if they are to be effective, he does grant that familiarity has a strengthening influence. The following findings of Katona also deserve mention : Ideal colour-constancy was attained with many objects and many observers. The colour-constancy of a figure is much greater than that of a ground. In agreement with my own earlier discussion, Katona finds that movement enhances colour-constancy. If colour-constancy is to appear at all, there must be, according to Katona, at least two illuminations of one object or two objects in one illumination. In making this formulation, Katona approaches very closely the views advanced by Mintz and Gelb. In spite of the importance which articulation of the visual field has for colour-constancy, I cannot attribute to it an all-important or even a decisive significance.

---

[1] This does not depend upon any recognition of forms.

Mintz[1] has also reported a number of observations showing a certain dependence of the impression of illumination, and hence of the degree of colour-constancy, upon the articulation of the visual field. The severance of illumination and illuminated object is determined by " totality properties of the visual field and of its parts " or by "factors similar to those determining the phenomenal articulation and organization of the visual field." " The colour of the illumination and of the illuminated object, i.e., the illumination colour and the object colour, are accordingly particular aspects of the perception of total properties of the visual field. So-called transformation phenomena thus exemplify a determination of aspects of perception by the total configuration." Although field articulation undoubtedly has an influence upon colour-constancy, Mintz's generalization is hardly justified.

Finally, we shall discuss the views developed by Gelb, whose position is close to that of Mintz. Gelb's starting-point is an experiment of Bühler's to be described in greater detail below (§ 63). Gelb closes his criticism of this experiment with these words : " At least two surfaces of different albedo must be present in the visual field if there is to be a severance of illumination and illuminated object." [2] Gelb also describes the following experiment : " We set up a velvet-black disc on a colour-wheel in a half-darkened room . . . and concentrated the light of an arc-lamp upon it in such a way that the bounding rays of the cone of light coincided as sharply as possible with the edge of the disc. . . . When the black disc was rotated, it appeared white or whitish grey and in that (perceived) illumination or spatial brightness which was prevalent in the rest of the weakly illuminated room. This impression of white is absolutely compelling. . . . It also makes no difference whether we look at the disc from its immediate neighbourhood or from a greater distance. . . . The impression is suddenly changed, however, as soon as we introduce a piece of really white paper,

[1] A. Mintz, *Psychol. Forsch.*, 1928, 10.   [2] Gelb, p. 674.

however small it may be, into the path of the rays from the arc-lamp, at a distance of a few centimetres before the rotating disc ; at this very moment, we see the disc as black, the small piece of paper as white, and both as intensely illuminated. . . . When we remove the small piece of white paper . . . the disc again appears white." This experiment, which is very impressive, is described quite accurately, but I do not believe that it justifies Gelb's general conclusion which I have set forth above. Even Gelb himself admits that the disc on the colour-wheel, when it is presented alone, appears in the weak illumination of the room, *i.e.*, some illumination is really perceptible even under these conditions. According to our view, we can understand immediately that it appears not black but brighter because it closely resembles film colour and appears to lie in a weakly illuminated space, but with considerable intrinsic light-intensity. The articulation of the visual field does not create the impression of illumination, but can only strengthen it and thereby heighten the degree of colour-constancy. As soon as the small paper is introduced, the brighter and darker surfaces become organized and merge into a figural unity, *viz.*, into a field appearing in unitary illumination. Within this unitary field the impression of illumination and of illuminated colours is determined by certain factors to be mentioned later—primarily, the degrees of distinctness of material structure, and the insistence of the field (§ 65). The condition of double articulation which is given by Gelb, Mintz and Katona as a condition for the perception of illumination is neither necessary nor sufficient. Even a colour filling the entire visual field may appear with a distinct impression of illumination, as, for instance, the interesting observations of Metzger in connection with the total field have shown. " Usually we see in the total field not mere light but an illuminated area having a particular phenomenal spatial brightness. Object colour and illumination are not so clearly severed here, however, as when we see space filled with objects. Under various intensities of illumination, we do not always see simply the same unmodified object colour 'white' in various illuminations, nor do we always see merely a change in the object colour. The two are changed, but not exactly in parallel fashion, and in any particular case it is very difficult to make separate reports about the components."[1] If illumination and illuminated object are to be seen simultaneously in the total field, at least a trace of microstructure must be present; visibility of boundary lines is not in itself sufficient. "The texture of the objective surface, *even if it lie below the limen of visibility*, is the principal factor in the formation of a phenomenal surface."[2] I do not believe that microstructure can immediately be set, phenomenologically and genetically, on par with those macrostructures which contribute to an inner organization of the visual field. What we have said demonstrates that a double articulation of the visual field is *unnecessary* for the impression of illumination. This same condition is also in itself *insufficient*, as the following observation shows. If the coloured fields in a Weber photometer are different, there is a distinct double articulation of the visual field, or, if we add the boundary, a triple articulation; but we cannot speak properly of any experience of illumination in this field.

Finally we shall discuss briefly attempts to introduce into our field of investigation Wertheimer's law of precision (*Prägnanz*), which has led to such interesting discussions in the realm of figures. In the field of colour, the law is interpreted as an original tendency toward precision of colour-matter. In their study cited above, Gelb and Granit have taken the first step in this direction. "The fact that the limen for a figural field is greater than the limen for a ground field illustrates a general law, *viz.*, the tendency toward the formation of configurations which are as simple and as precisely defined as possible—or the tendency toward precision of configuration, in Wertheimer's sense. . . . Since lack of homogeneity in colouring impairs the precision of the

---

[1] Metzger, I, p. 6.   [2] *Ibid.*, p. 13.

figural fields which we have used, there is a tendency for them to appear as homogeneous as possible, and hence the colour-limen for figural fields lies higher, in our experiments, than for equally bright ground fields."[1] This experiment of Gelb and Granit has, however, met with contradiction. G. E. Müller has shown that we should not speak of precision of a colour in the sense here intended, even though the concept of precision may be applicable to forms.[2] Ackermann raises the following objection : " Even if the infield has the most clear-cut *figural* character, it is by no means completely indifferent to small additions of colour." He found that even small additions of colour to a well-defined white caused an immediate effect.[3] In a critical review of Granit's study cited above, I myself had occasion to set forth my views on the law of precision as applied to colours. Like Wertheimer, Granit finds his point of departure in the view that " seen objects strive for formal precision ; a seen multiplicity of objects does not ordinarily appear in confused juxtaposition, but is organized by an inner spontaneous activity according to certain laws of totality ; there is under all conditions an inner tendency toward precision of configuration." When this is applied to his own experiments, Granit believes that it means that " the given physical stimuli are not the only determiners of the impression ; rather, the figure will always assume the colour which permits its form to emerge most clearly. We are not presupposing here a free creation of something entirely new, but simply a particular kind of use of the given stimuli in the direction of greater precision." Granit attempts to show, by particular examples, why it is " meaningful " for a figure in one case to assume one colour and in another case another colour. In my review I have shown that the law of precision, which may do good service in connection with the perception of figures, has here been transferred to an inappropriate field. The

---

[1] Gelb and Granit, p. 105.
[2] *Zsch. f. Psychol.*, 1925, 97, p. 347.
[3] *Psychol. Forsch.*, 1924, 5.

effect of this tendency toward precision in the former cases, where it has long been recognized, is completely different from what it is in the latter. If several luminous points which do not really lie in a circular path appear to be laid in a form resembling a circle, we note a tendency for the circular form to be preferred in perception. We may not succeed at all, or may not succeed to the same extent, in perceiving the pattern as a circle if the conditions of observation are made more favourable, *e.g.*, if tachistoscopic exposition is replaced by longer exposition, or if the illumination is made general. Under favourable conditions, we apprehend the true non-circular arrangement of the luminous points. In Granit's experiments, the tendency toward precision of configuration would be acting under convenient and natural conditions and not, as in the early observations of the *gestalt* psychologists, under difficult conditions of observation. Granit's view is also contradicted by the fact that the degree of colour-constancy is reduced in tachistoscopic exposition. Until such contradictions are completely resolved, we should be cautious in applying the general principle of precision to colour-constancy.

§ 32. Memory Colours

We shall explain briefly our attitude toward Hering's memory colours.[1] " The colour in which we have most often seen an external object is imprinted indelibly upon our memory and becomes a fixed property of the memory-image." Hering calls this colour the " memory colour " of the object. " Just as the memory colour of an object is always called up when a memory-image of the object is aroused by one of its other attributes or even simply by the word by which we name the object, it is aroused with particular force when we see the object again or even think that we are seeing it, and it then determines the way in which we see it." Hering makes the tacit assumption that we see external objects most of the time in

[1] Hering, VI, p. 7 f.

normal illumination. We might say, then, that the memory colours of familiar objects are those colours in which the objects are seen under normal illumination. I should prefer this definition of memory colours to Hering's. Since in everyday life normal illumination is also the prevalent illumination, we can hardly decide in favour of one definition or the other simply by considering the usual cases in which memory colours have been developed. Yet the memory colour of an object, which never appears except under *non-normal* illumination, should represent approximately the colour of the object seen *in normal illumination.*

If an object to which we ascribe a memory colour is lying in normal illumination, the actual colour-impression agrees perfectly with the memory colour of the object. If it is not in normal illumination, the memory colour determines the nature of what we see more than does the " genuine " colour of an object which has no memory colour. Under otherwise identical conditions, a memory colour can exercise an even stronger influence upon colour-vision. If I am to see as " white " a white paper standing in reduced illumination, I must be able to survey clearly its conditions of illumination. If that is impossible, I see the white paper rather as if it were reduced to normal illumination. The situation is different if the object has a pronounced memory colour. Even if the conditions are such that I cannot adequately survey the conditions of illumination, but are such that I am able to recognize it as a familiar object of known memory colour, this memory colour may have a strong influence upon vision. Over against the stronger effect of memory colours stands the greater lability of the colour-impressions formed under their influence.[1] I have often made the following pertinent observation while walking. I hold pieces of paper in such a way that they " frame " a distant meadow or a portion of green field, whose colours are strongly influenced by aerial perspective. I can still perceive the distance fairly well, but since surrounding

---

[1] *Cf.* § 33.

L

objects are covered, I cannot recognize what objects I am seeing in the frame. I cannot recognize the genuine colours of these objects enclosed in the frame, but as soon as I remove the frame and perceive that distant strip as a meadow or green field, its memory colour comes into play and I believe that I can perceive distinctly the green of the meadow and the brown of the soil. We shall not go astray if we ascribe to the naturally coloured objects which we encounter most frequently (snow, blood, coal, plants) memory colours which are similar for all individuals with normal colour-vision. Objects, such as articles of clothing, which are seen especially by their owners, develop memory colours only for these individuals. In practical life it is only through " surprises " that we realize clearly the effects of memory colours. Matthaei has described such a case. He saw quite distinctly in a poorly illuminated photograph the natural chromatic colours of the objects represented, but this chromatic colouring proved to be illusory when the photograph was brought into good light.[1]

Memory colours play no rôle in any of the quantitative experiments of the present work, for the papers which were exposed for judgment neither had any particular individuality nor were familiar to the observers. I may add that it is impossible, or at least very difficult, to arrange quantitative experiments with memory colours on account of their peculiar lability, as the above-mentioned observation of Matthaei shows.

There are many indications that there exist, in addition to the more or less permanent memory colours of which we have just spoken, others which arise momentarily under particular visual attitudes and have only a fleeting existence. Fuchs [2] cites the following observation made by Helmholtz : [3] if a blue shadow is produced upon a white background by candle-light, it persists after it has developed clearly, even if we remove the objective cause

---

[1] Matthaei, p. 310.   [2] Fuchs, I, p. 193.
[3] *Physiol. Optik*, 3rd ed., vol 2, p. 231.

by extinguishing the candle. Fuchs likewise refers to an
inversion experiment by Mach,[1] which shows that colours
which have been brought about by inversion do not
disappear immediately when the inversion vanishes.
Fuchs reports still other similar observations. I myself
can give the following contribution. I have described
above [2] the experiment by Gelb in which a black paper
lighted by an arc-light actually appeared black only
when a small piece of white paper was in the field. For
me, the black paper remains distinctly black for some time
after the white paper has been removed. In all of these
cases we might very well appeal to temporary memory
colours owing their origin to special visual attitudes.

> The only theory of colour-constancy in which memory colour
> plays a significant rôle is that of Kaila. " Let us suppose that
> the visual organ has learned, on the basis of memory colours, to
> segregate the process corresponding to the colour of the illumina-
> tion from the local processes corresponding to object colours,
> and has thus learned to effect that peculiar and puzzling splitting
> of colour-sensations into anomalous (phenomenal) illuminations
> and real surface colours. It is then reasonable to assume that
> this splitting can be achieved by the visual organ even when no
> memory colours stand at its disposal." [3]

When the colour of an object rises above the normal
in brightness, darkness or saturation, language tends to
exaggerate almost immeasurably the actual overstepping
of the norm. There are striking examples of this not only
in poetry (" as white as snow," " as red as blood," " as
black as ebony," " a jet-black negro ") but also in ordinary
language, which is also prone to exaggerate, especially
when colour-names release affective ideas (" a face as
white as chalk " or " as red as a beet "). We note, if
not an exaggeration, at least a marked *emphasizing* of
colour-attributes in our tendency to name colours
according to the attributes which are most striking in
actual perception. When we are looking at two fabrics,

[1] *Analyse der Empfindungen*, 4th ed., p. 162.
[2] *Cf.* p. 90.
[3] Kaila, *Psychol. Forsch.*, 1923, 3, p. 51.

one of which has a bluish and the other a brownish component, we are likely to neglect their other colour-attributes, such as brightness, and speak of the materials as simply " blue " and " brown." There seems to be a certain relationship between the exaggeration of colour-attributes in language and the fact that in imagination we exaggerate colours of objects whose colours are generally distinguished only in terms of brightness, darkness or hue. If we ask a person to pick out a blue which will match the colour of the eyes of someone he knows very well, he generally selects a blue which is too saturated. If we ask a person to match the black of his hat, the red of his lips or the colour of a brick, he usually chooses a black which is too deep or reds which are too highly saturated. Almost always he selects a colour which is too bright to match a bright object, one which is too dark to match a dark object, and one which is too saturated to match an object which is known to have a distinct hue. A reflective attitude must be avoided in these matchings. Exaggeration is most easily demonstrated in naïve adults and in children. The form of language transmitted to the child has great significance for his thinking and imagination ; exaggeration of attributes of memory colours may be determined as much by language (description of colours in fairy stories, etc.) as by individual perception itself. Originally, the absolute strikingness of the whiteness, blackness or hue of certain objects may have led to an exaggeration of these colour-attributes in memory. Saturated colours are extremely rare in nature, and we hardly ever encounter pronounced whites or deep blacks except in artificially coloured objects. We hardly ever see white as a natural colour except in snow. *As a rule, the exaggeration in language of colour-peculiarities of objects and their imprints in memory are results of the absolute striking character of these colour-peculiarities.*

In art, colour is used either for ornament and decoration or for purposes of representing nature. It is often impossible, however, to carry through this simple distinction in various fields of art. Frequently colour has a decorative purpose even when it is serving more particularly to represent nature. Hence it is not alone in paintings which attempt to imitate nature that we find an exaggerated saturation of local colours; high saturation is, rather, a general rule. It is interesting to speculate whether it may not be the exaggeration of hues of familiar objects (eyes, lips, etc.) in pictures which influences the formation of the memory colours of these objects in the way described.

Sometimes attempts have been made to deduce the brilliant character of the paintings of the old masters from their lack of consideration of the changes which colours undergo as a result of light and shade, air and distance; it is, however, impossible to ascribe the exaggerated saturation of the chromatic colours which represent objects in " normal " illumination (and such illumination prevails in those pictures) to a failure to take illumination into account. A normal illumination does not cause chromatic colours to appear in exaggerated saturation. The exaggeration of colours in the art of painting serves, primarily, decorative needs.

Both shadowing and lighting make the finer structure of the surfaces of objects unrecognizable and may thus, to a certain degree, obscure their " materiality." The illumination-scale of Leonardo da Vinci extends from the deep darkness of shadows only to the brightness of normal illumination, although in his book on painting he describes in detail the changes which colours undergo in sunlight and in artificial light. In his book he also expresses preference for full daylight above other intensities of illumination for purposes of painting.[1] When we are demonstrating an object for purposes of instruction, we show it, if possible, in normal daylight. We must bear this in mind if we wish to understand the method of painting of the old masters. They are above all narrators, seeking to set before the observer men and things in all

---

[1] Leonardo da Vinci, *Das Buch der Malerei*. Translated by H. Ludwig. Text and translation. Vol. I. Wien, 1882, pp. 145, 155.

their natural characteristics ; they are more interested in *what they are representing* than in solving " problems of painting." For these reasons, normal daylight illumination prevails in their pictures, and their colours are almost always normally illuminated. Wherever the modelling of objects necessitates a representation of shaded parts, the shading is not taken fully into account and colours are painted too much *in the direction of genuine colours.* The *qualitative* modifications of colours (the " deepening " of hues) which keep pace with reduction of illumination are seldom recognized. A shadow is represented by shades of grey. The qualitative changes resulting from aerial perspective are underestimated. The way in which these painters represent conditions of illumination is very similar to tendencies in the selection of colours which we find in beginners in painting, who also grant local colours an unjustified influence upon colouring.

Quite gradually new means of expression were introduced into the art of painting. It was probably Giorgione who first successfully extended the realm of painting to illumination transcending the normal and also tried to reproduce " light " itself. The representation of light and shade was Rembrandt's main problem. In those works of Rembrandt in which his individuality is particularly expressed, we find that surface colours in normal illumination are almost entirely suppressed and function only as mediators between shading and lighting. Thus we see almost all the colours of his paintings only through light and shade.

I am convinced that exact analyses of colour-perception will make possible a fruitful investigation of the painter's means of expression ; up to this time we have only insignificant approaches to such a study. A rich field of research is here opened for experimental æsthetics. " Æsthetics from below," in so far as it deals with colours, can hope to approach its goal—that of making a picture æsthetically intelligible—only when it turns to a consideration of the whole world of colour-phenomena.

Studies in experimental æsthetics will thereby come into closer contact with art itself.[1]

§ 33. SUBJECTIVE AND OBJECTIVE ATTITUDES

Hering [2] notes incidentally that a memory colour can completely determine vision " provided that we do not attend particularly to the colour." We may generalize this observation of Hering's. Whenever we are attempting to recognize the colour of an object, it is disadvantageous to attend to the colour-phenomena themselves and neglect the coloured object. Such an attitude agrees essentially with the attitude often called " critical." Gelb speaks of an attitude which is relatively distant from reality and which he calls an " attitude of pure optics " ; Köhler has remarked incidentally that this attitude causes us " to free ourselves from the object-character of the surfaces and degrade them into mere extents of light." [3] Not all the products of colour-perception with which we are dealing in this work are impaired to the same extent by this subjective attitude. Its effect is most obvious when memory colours play a part. What we have just seen as the green of a distant mountain meadow becomes transformed into an entirely different colour (difficult to characterize more exactly) when we begin to submerge ourselves in the colour-phenomenon itself and to disregard the object as a part of the landscape. The disturbing effect of this subjective attitude is also very noticeable in the case of " shaded " and " lighted " surface colours. A subjective attitude toward such colour-impressions causes them to become more similar to the colours appearing after reduction (to the prevailing illumination of the visual field). The disturbing effect of this attitude also appears, in a slight degree, in connection with surface colours lying in a section of the visual field in which

[1] Cf. D. Katz, " Experimentelle Psychologie und Gemäldekunst," 5. Kong. f. exper. Psychol., Leipzig, 1912 ; D. Katz, " Psychologisches zur Frage der Farbengebung," 1. Kong. f. Aesthetik u. allg. Kunstwissen., Stuttgart, 1914.
[2] Hering, VI, p. 8.   [3] Gelb, p. 599 f.

illumination is generally reduced or heightened. In these cases, the colours appear to be modified in the direction toward which they would be shifted by reduction to normal illumination. A white paper lying in a remote part of a room appears darker with " subjective " direction of attention than with free inspection of the paper as an object. We must emphasize, however, that neither in the latter case nor in the cases of shading and lighting does the subjective attitude ever cause colours to appear exactly as they would after reduction to normal illumination. Surface colours in a uniformly and normally illuminated visual field prove to be nearly invariable as attention is variously directed.

The attitude which we have called " subjective " is far removed from the natural attitude of everyday life. It is sometimes adopted by the psychologist in his experiments, although it does not become habitual to him. Presumably, however, it should be dominant in the painter. If one is a psychologist and painter at the same time, the subjective attitude may become so compelling that he is no longer able to perceive certain phenomena of colour-constancy. We need not discuss here again the vision of the painter, for we have already said what is necessary. It should be clear from those discussions that all of our results concerning the modification of colour-phenomena by a subjective attitude may easily be understood in terms of tendencies toward reduced vision (*i.e.*, vision reduced to the prevalent illumination) which arise from this attitude.

It seems important to mention that when we are attempting to see reductively without a reduction-screen, our eye-movements are different from those involved in normal vision. Whereas in normal perception we tend to move our eyes over the centres of the surfaces, in reductive vision we carry them to the boundary contours between the variously illuminated areas.

It seems possible to demonstrate inhibitory influence of the subjective attitude upon colours differing in their modes of appearance from surface colours. I always perceive a loss of lustre, for example, when I turn to the colour-phenomenon itself and do not consider so much the lustrous *object*. The impressions of volume colour and transparency are also most distinct in unbiassed observation directed toward the objects themselves.

§ 34. COLOUR-CONSTANCY AND MONOCULAR VISION

In the experiments in which the exposition-time was shortened, we attributed the resulting tendencies toward reduced vision to a less precise apprehension of spatial relationships. If this explanation is correct, we should also find reductive tendencies in other situations in which apprehension of spatial relationships is inhibited. We should note such a tendency, for example, when we replace binocular by monocular vision. A brightly coloured wall, weakly illuminated by daylight or artificial light and located far from a window, gives distinctly different impressions of brightness in monocular and in binocular vision. If I shift from binocular to monocular vision, the wall is darkened. If I first look monocularly and then binocularly, the *brightening* is rather more distinct than is the *darkening* in the opposite case. We hardly need to say that such changes in colour appearing when we pass from monocular to binocular vision are not to be brought into connection with those which we observe in Fechner's paradoxical experiment.[1]

In connection with our experiments in which the exposition-time was varied, we performed others on the brightening of normally illuminated colours through binocular observation. The experiments with the exposition-time t_4 were repeated with monocular observation.

OBSERVER K

Binocular observation	Value II	Disc $B_1 = 56 \cdot 4°$ W
Monocular ,,	,, II	,, $B_1 = 23 \cdot 2°$ W
	B Values	Q Values
Binocular ,,	$0 \cdot 17$	$4 \cdot 0$
Monocular ,,	$0 \cdot 08$	$1 \cdot 9$

[1] Fechner, " Ueber einige Verhältnisse des binokularen Sehens," *Abhandl. d. math.-phys. Kl. d. kgl. sächs. Ges. d. Wiss.*, 1861, 5, p. 416 ff.

Observer *P*

Binocular observation	Value II	Disc $B_1 = 92 \cdot 9°$ W
Monocular ,,	,, II	,, $B_1 = 54 \cdot 8°$ W

	B Values	*Q* Values
Binocular ,,	0·27	6·4
Monocular ,,	0·15	3·9

We note that colour-constancy is considerably lower in monocular observation. The quotient *Q*, which characterizes the brightening, is, for both observers, only about half as great in monocular as in binocular observation. We have not attempted here to measure quantitatively the decrease of colour-constancy in monocular observation for colours under other conditions ; we shall have occasion to do this later in connection with other experiments. Our experiments have disclosed the fact that the double eye functions to ensure colour-constancy in a higher degree than does the single eye.

This function of the double eye might be explained in terms of the superior apprehension of *spatial* relations in binocular vision. The increase in the reality-character of perceived objects in binocular vision is most intimately interwoven with this fact, and this always acts, as we have seen, in the direction of higher colour-constancy.[1]

It is so obvious that lustre is more distinct in binocular than in monocular vision that sometimes the very existence of monocular lustre has been questioned. Volume colours are distinct only in binocular observation—a fact which may very probably be explained in terms of better apprehension of spatial relationships in binocular vision. Glowing colours are perceived equally well in monocular and binocular vision. Incidentally it seems to follow from this, as we have already mentioned, that glow does not require voluminousness. The transparency of colours is strongly reduced in monocular observation.

[1] Hornbostel has recognized certain similarities between monocular vision and monaural hearing on the one hand and binocular vision and binaural hearing on the other. If we close one ear, a noise becomes less full, thick and stable ; it becomes less sharp, decisive and *objective*. E. v. Hornbostel, *Handb. d. norm. u. pathol., Physiologie*, 11, 1926.

When a painter is trying to apprehend the colour-values to be placed upon the canvas, he bends over or looks under his arm at the landscape in order not to be influenced by the " genuine " colours of the objects. This disturbs his survey of the conditions of illumination and makes recognition of objects difficult ; a relatively reduced vision is the result. We may act in a similar way if we wish to suppress the precise perception of orientation and localization of coloured surfaces and the related colour-constancy. An observer reaches this goal, for example, when he bends his head markedly to the side or looks at a situation through a plane mirror which causes it to appear turned through a certain angle from its true position.

§ 35. COLOUR-CONSTANCY AND PUPILLARY ADJUSTMENT

Of two achromatic film colours or surface colours in equal illumination, the brighter colour has the greater pupillo-motor effect. Now what can be said about the pupillo-motor valences of two colour-impressions based upon the same retinal excitations but appearing subjectively as different ? Is the pupillo-motor valence a function only of the impinging light or also of the subjective impression of brightness ? Naturally this question is justified, since, as we know, the activity of the pupils is not generally free from psychic influences. We may recall O. Haab's cortical reflex of the pupil. We remember also that according to J. Piltz, even imagining black and white objects may have as a result certain changes in the size of the pupils.[1] We might expect, therefore, that changes in perception might influence the behaviour of the pupil, even with the same retinal excitation.

Set-up II [2] was used for a series of experiments directed toward this problem. The dimensions of the discs *A* and *B* were the same as before. Since the problem was

[1] O. Schwarz calls these two reflexes cortical light-reflexes. *Die Funktionsprüfung des Auges.* Berlin, 1904, p. 214.

[2] *Cf.* p. 95.

not to measure the absolute magnitude of the diameters of the pupils but only to discover any changes that might occur during alternate inspection of discs A and B, I sat by the side of the observer and observed the behaviour of the pupils directly.

Experiment (a). We set up 360° W on disc A; disc B was equated to it in *quality*. When the eye moved from A to B, there was a narrowing of the pupil. With reversed movement, the pupil dilated somewhat less.

Experiment (b). We set up 360° W on disc A, and disc B was so set that it reflected the same amount of light as A. When the eye moved from A to B and then back, no changes in the pupil could be observed. We hardly need to say that with these settings the discs appeared subjectively as very different—A as a light grey and B as a blackish grey. We noted distinct movements of the pupils, however, when we showed the observer two papers in equally strong (*e.g.*, normal) illumination and with a brightness-difference of this magnitude.

Our experiments suggest this generalization: The pupillo-motor valences of surface colours in illuminations of different intensities are determined by the intensities of the accompanying retinal processes and appear to be essentially independent of central factors.

CHAPTER II

Chromatic Surface Colours in Various Illuminations

§ 36. MODIFICATIONS OF CHROMATIC SURFACE COLOUR

THE brightness of a chromatic surface colour is generally defined in terms of its correspondence to a particular member of the black-white series. Using a scale of greys, we ascertained, in normal illumination, the brightness-values of a large series of chromatic colour-squares differing widely in saturation. Our method was that described by F. Hillebrand.[1] I replaced the colour-wheel carrying disc B_2 in the apparatus described above [2] by a holder of white cardboard, with its upper edge somewhat inclined away from the observer but standing essentially in a vertical position ; in each individual case one of the chromatic·squares and the equally bright achromatic square were exposed upon it. The two squares were now observed through an episcotister and their brightnesses were compared. When we reduced the opening of the episcotister a few degrees to a point at which the squares were just perceptible, we found that the brightness equation made in normal illumination remained practically unchanged. We are led to this generalization : When the intensity of illumination is reduced by means of an episcotister, chromatic surface colours of any saturation and brightness undergo essentially the same losses in brightness as do the members of the black-white series to which they are equal in brightness in normal illumination. If now we increase rather than reduce the intensity of illumination of chromatic surface colours,

[1] F. Hillebrand, *Ber. d. Kais. Akad. d. Wiss. in Wien*, 89, Abt. 3, 1889, p. 101 ff.
[2] *Cf.* p. 104.

e.g., by illuminating them with sunlight, we are led to this conclusion : With an increase in the intensity of illumination, chromatic surface colours of any saturation and brightness undergo essentially the same increase in brightness as do the members of the black-white series to which they are equal in brightness in normal illumination.

It is well known that we ascribe to the four principal colours in their highest degrees of saturation different specific brightnesses, yellow having the highest and blue the lowest brightness, and red having a higher specific brightness than green. As our earlier experiments showed, the achromatic colours resembling white maintain their brightness more strongly when illumination is diminished than do those near black. We might suspect, then, that when illumination is reduced, saturated yellow will undergo relatively the least and saturated blue relatively the greatest loss in brightness. This expectation is confirmed by observation. If we look at a yellow and a blue paper, both of the highest possible saturation, through an episcotister with a small opening, yellow still seems to stand very near white, while the brightness of the blue has approached that of black to a marked degree.

In the following experiments, which dealt with the saturation of chromatic surface colours in non-normal illumination, we again used the apparatus described on p. 153. B_2 was a pale red disc, its brightness amounting to approximately $240° W$. The problem was to set up on B_1 a colour which was equal in saturation and brightness to the impression of B_2 as seen through an episcotister-opening of $5°$. The following values are arithmetic means of three settings :

> Observer C.
> $B_1 = 40° W$, $151° R$,[1] $169° B$.
> Observer D.
> $B_1 = 35° W$, $45° R$, $280° B$.
> Observer E.
> $B_1 = 50° W$, $94° R$, $216° B$.

---

[1] " R " refers to the pale red colour.

I expected that when B_2 was seen through an episco-tister-opening of 5°, it would be possible to perceive, at the most, only traces of red. This was not in the least the case, however, since the red was quite distinct. Its degree of saturation depends upon the setting of disc B_1.

We obtained corresponding values when we used other chromatic colours. We may conclude from the experiments that when we look through an episcotister at a surface colour which is intrinsically unsaturated, the colour undergoes only a slight loss in saturation. With an opening of 2°, *i.e.*, with a reduction of the chromatic lights to 1/180 of their normal values, a chromatic colour may still be apprehended. Now let us replace the unsaturated colours by colours of higher saturation. Then with an opening of the episcotister which still permits us to perceive the disc B_2 (about $\frac{1}{2}$°), the colours appear immediately in saturations lying above the limen and not significantly weaker than those of the same papers when they are seen directly. It is difficult to decide whether four colours resembling the principal colours undergo similar or different losses in saturation with the same opening of the episcotister. I pasted side by side four square papers of high saturation, brought them into the position of B_2 and made the opening of the episcotister about $\frac{3}{4}$°. Numerous observers then said, in close agreement with each other, that yellow was highest and blue lowest in saturation, and that the red and green, which were approximately the same in saturation, stood nearer to blue than to yellow.

We may formulate the results of our last experiments as follows : If we reduce very markedly the intensity of illumination of chromatic surface colours, they lose only slightly in saturation when they are seen by a light-adapted eye. If we lower the illumination to about 1/480 of the normal, yellow appears to undergo the slightest and blue the greatest loss in saturation, while green and red occupy intermediate positions.

Both in our earlier experiments and in these experiments with the episcotister we may neglect the very slight amount of light falling into the eye from the episcotister-disc itself. Therefore we may make direct inferences from the size of the opening of the epicotister to the corresponding weakening of the chromatic lights from B_2 impinging upon the retina. We found that chromatic surface colours, seen through the episcotister, appeared in high saturation, in spite of the minimal intensity of the stimuli ; therefore there is a heightening of the chromatic components, just as there was a brightening or darkening of surface colours observed through the episcotister in the experiments reported above.

How may we characterize the difference which persists between the colour-impressions of discs B_1 and B_2, even though they are approximately the same in hue, saturation and brightness ? When the observers were asked this question, they were most inclined to characterize the difference as a difference in intensity or pronouncedness. It seems advisable to use here the terms which we applied to similar differences in the episcotister experiments with achromatic surface colours. We might then say that any two of the corresponding settings of B_1 and B_2 *represent two different degrees of pronouncedness of the same chromatic colour.*

According to our results, it is *impossible* to represent all surface colours by means of a tridimensional structure. Our studies show that *we can change any surface colour not only in three but in four independent directions.* In addition to changes in hue, brightness and saturation (which are possible even with *constant* illumination), we find changes toward other degrees of pronouncedness when the intensity of illumination is changed.

These relationships may be demonstrated graphically by means of various geometric constructions. We might represent the continuum of all surface colours appearing *in one particular intensity of illumination* by means of a double pyramid (or a similar figure) ; then the entire system of surface colours might be represented by as many such double pyramids or similar figures as there are distinguishable degrees of illumination.

§ 37. LIGHT AND DARK ADAPTATION AND THE CONSTANCY OF COLOUR

Hering was the first to propound the theory that contrast represents only a special expression of a more general principle of the functioning of the visual organ, *viz.*, the interaction between retinal elements. " Adaptation of the eye to light, which is dependent upon this interaction . . . appears almost immediately when illumination is changed ; hence I have called it *simultaneous* or instantaneous adaptation." [1] We must make a sharp distinction between such instantaneous adaptation and durative adaptation, since the two types of adaptation have entirely different causes and also significantly different effects. When dark adaptation sets in, the interaction of the elements in the visual field does not cease suddenly. Thus instantaneous and durative adaptation are continually overlapping.

We owe much to Noldt [2] for his investigation of instantaneous adaptation in which he varied extensively the intensities of the inducing and stimulus lights.

If we consider the capacity of the eye to recognize colours in different intensities of illumination, we are led to a stricter distinction between instantaneous and durative adaptation. We found that the colours of chromatic papers appear in approximately the same degrees of saturation after light adaptation as in normal illumination, and in their specific brightnesses, even when the intensity of the stimulus is minimal. Thus the light-adapted eye manifests a high degree of ability in recognizing chromatic colours under marked changes of intensity of illumination. When we are dark adapted, the Purkinje phenomenon disturbs recognition of colours in our environment ; it leads us astray in regard to the hue, saturation and brightness of the coloured objects around us, for we ascribe to the objects as their *genuine colours* those which they show in normal illumination to

[1] Hering, VI, p. 18. [2] *Zsch. f. Psychol.*, 1925, 97.

M

the light-adapted eye. The dark-adapted eye deceives us not only in regard to *chromatic* colours ; as a result of increase in its sensitivity, it may even deceive us in regard to the brightness of *achromatic* colours. If two lights of different intensity are seen under different degrees of dark adaptation, they may appear subjectively alike, or even the less intense light may appear to be more intense. Instantaneous adaptation may cause two lights of different intensity to appear more similar in their brightness, but never causes them to appear equally bright.

Results of studies of visual acuity demand a sharper functional distinction between the light-adapted and the dark-adapted eye. S. Bloom and S. Garten have shown that " the light-adapted eye may be even superior to the dark-adapted eye in visual acuity if the illumination of the test-cards (equally strong for the two eyes) is reduced to such a point that it does not blind the dark-adapted eye but permits the test-cards to appear moderately bright, while it lies far below the illumination which is most favourable for the visual acuity of the light-adapted eye." [1] Since I suspected that it was the *high visual acuity of the light-adapted eye* which might cause the superiority of the light-adapted eye over the dark-adapted ·eye in colour-recognition, I tested the statement of Bloom and Garten by means of an apparatus described above (p. 104). First I decreased the opening of the episcotister to a point at which printing seen through it could still be read easily with a light-adapted eye. This was possible with an opening of about $\frac{1}{4}^{\circ}$. After fifteen or twenty minutes of dark adaptation, the printing became scarcely visible, or even invisible, with the same opening of the episcotister. This confirmed the statement of Bloom and Garten cited above. What is particularly interesting in this connection is the fact that for the dark-adapted eye there is no longer an impression of a surface of white paper with black letters. The surface as a whole seems perhaps more insistent to the dark-adapted eye (even *blinding* to some observers), but it never becomes

---

[1] *Pflügers Arch.*, 1907, 72.

really *whiter*; the extended area has no longer the mode
of appearance of surface colour but shows, rather, a
certain similarity to film colour. Its illumination seems
to be of an unusual kind, in so far as we may speak of
illumination at all.

Since the reduction of visual acuity also reduces
distinctness of microstructure, the loss of clear-cut surface
colours under dark adaptation should not surprise us. We
must assume that *pronounced surface colours are formed only
with the co-operation of the cone-apparatus. The mode of
appearance which is mediated by the rods resembles film
colour.*[1] The duplicity of the visual organ is thus revealed
even in the difference between the modes of appearance
of colours corresponding to its two mechanisms for
perception of light. It is also noteworthy that the
impression of *luminosity* persists even in complete dark
adaptation. Objects which give the impression of lustre
to the light-adapted eye appear luminous to the dark-
adapted eye, if the intensity of the light is suitable;
they may cause a *weird luminosity* on the periphery of the
dark-adapted eye.

Estimates of the degree of colour-constancy present in
dark adaptation cannot be made by means of an immediate comparison of colours presented in a dark field
with colours presented in a light field. All that we can
do is to undertake absolute judgments with the dark-
adapted eye. I found Burzlaff's colour-chart quite
suitable for this purpose. After a half-hour of dark
adaptation, the observer looked at this chart in a dark-
room in very weak illumination. We found an extensive
simplification of the chart; most steps distinguishable by
the light-adapted eye had vanished and altogether there
remained only three qualities, almost immediately adjacent
to each other, these being white, dark grey and black,
and dark grey occupying the most space. The white
was still a distinct white, even though it was very unpronounced; the black was likewise distinct. The dark

---

[1] G. E. Müller speaks of a " spatial " mode of appearance of rod colours.
Zsch. f. Sinnesphysiol., 1923, 54, p. 140 f.

grey had the unpronounced character of subjective grey. It is difficult to specify numerical limits for these three colour-regions ; we may indicate approximate limits by saying that the " white " region extended to about 236° W and that the " black " region began with about 48° W. This decrease in the number of colour-steps in the black-white series suggests a marked decrease in colour-constancy, even for achromatic colours, during dark adaptation.

Walker's[1] experiments on the shadowing of surface colours lead him to conclude that colour-constancy is higher in eidetic adults than in non-eidetic adults. The values which he gives to support this conclusion are not entirely convincing, since the reported differences lie within the range of inter-individual and intra-individual differences found elsewhere. Walker maintains that colour-constancy reaches its highest point in the years just before puberty, but this statement does not seem to be completely justified by the values given, and even if it were, it would be difficult to draw from it the conclusions at which Walker arrives. " The maximum of brightness-transformation, as well as the maximum of dark adaptation, is found in the eidetic age. . . . That should furnish proof for the view that the two phenomena belong together " (p. 377). If this conclusion does not seem to me to be entirely justified, the following one is still less so : " Our proof that simultaneous contrast and transformation belong together should be firmly established through our discovery of heightened and psychically integrated phenomena of adaptation " (p. 380). It is remarkable that in the entire study we can find nothing concerning experiments on contrast ! " We shall thus have to assume that phenomena of transformation persist as results of the heightened and psychically integrated adaptation of the early phase of development " (p. 383). Against this conclusion we may bring many arguments, of which I shall mention only the following. In their studies of perception of illumination, the members of the Marburg group seem to be dominated by the view,

[1] W. Walker, *Zsch. f. Psychol.*, 1927, 103.

untenable on phenomenological grounds, that processes of adaptation lead to a kind of elimination of illumination ; but such an adjustment—we must repeat—is out of the question. This is a keystone of the Marburg position ; if it is dislodged, all of the statements about the explanation of colour-constancy which are supported by it become doubtful. " An illumination colour is really *neutralized* in phenomena of transformation ; for it is discounted immediately in any case and becomes an extremely unpronounced and unsaturated colour which, in general, cannot be compared with an otherwise similar colour." This is the most recent formulation of Jaensch's position to which we can refer.[1] I cannot accept his view. An illumination colour is not neutralized as an illumination colour ; on the contrary, it is very distinct and creates that characteristic impression of illumination without which the phenomena presented in every illuminated visual field would not exist at all. It would be not at all desirable, so to say, for adaptation to eradicate illumination colour, for adaptation has a result opposed to the degree of distinctness of the phenomena of illumination. The more complete adaptation is, the less the specific phenomena of illumination could appear.

It is difficult to bring into accord with Walker's view the fact that in dark adaptation the colour-constancy of the normal individual reaches its lowest point for achromatic colour and is entirely lost for chromatic colours and chromatic illumination. Also I fail to see any place in Walker's theory for the facts of colour-constancy in animals, unless it be that even fish, for example, are provided with eidetic phenomena or have passed through an eidetic stage. Finally, Walker's theory makes it hard to understand the fact that we have been able to find even in five-year-old children an almost ideal degree of colour-constancy, agreeing with that of adults (§ 60).

According to Brunswik's experiments, the relationships between colour-constancy and eidetic disposition are not

[1] E. R. Jaensch, *Ueber Grundfragen der Farbenpsychologie*. Leipzig, 1930, p. 457.

as simple as Walker assumes.[1]   Brunswik suspects that
the relationships between the eidetic constitution and
colour-constancy are only indirect.   He points out that
strong eidetics frequently show high colour-constancy.
We shall return in § 61 to the relationships between
eidetic imagery and colour-constancy.

Jaensch and Stallmann [2] consider that rod-vision is only
a special case of an older (primordial) type of vision.
Relying upon findings by Hess,[3] Katz and Révész,[4] and
Reichner,[5] they maintain that even the cones can mediate
primordial vision.   " Functioning of the cones and their
correlates in the central nervous system must be included
among the external conditions of twilight vision, and
functioning of the rods among those of daylight vision "
(p. 140).   According to Jaensch,[6] the Purkinje phenomenon
" may appear without functioning of the rods as an
expression of a purely functional state of the neural sector
of the visual organ."   We are told that the coupling of
form-vision with a particular distribution of brightness
of the light-adapted eye is not anatomically conditioned ;
Jaensch believes rather " that the functional coupling is
of *primary* significance and that the functions immediately
promote each other, belong together and are unified "
(p. 249).   " The function is primary and has created the
structure of the organs " (p. 250).   Now, according to
Jaensch, the double function of the eye is adjusted to
perception of light and shadow in daylight vision, but not
to twilight vision.   Schrödinger and numerous other
investigators are of the opinion that the rods are adapted
to twilight vision in water.   " The rod-apparatus is an
. . . older visual organ which arose at the time of life
in the water." [7]   Jaensch rejects this theory.   " In view
of the high degree of plasticity and adaptability demonstrable at least in man, it is entirely improbable that
primitive adaptations which have now become meaningless

[1] *Zsch. f. Psychol.*, 1928, 109.   [2] *Ibid.*, 106.
[3] C. v. Hess, *Vergleichende Physiologie des Gesichtssinnes.* Jena, 1912.
[4] *Zsch. f. Psychol.*, 1909, 50.   [5] *Ibid.*, 1924, 96.
[6] E. Jaensch, *Zsch. f. Psychol.*, 1928, 106.
[7] E. Schrödinger, *Die Naturwissenschaften*, Jahrg. 1924, p. 927.

would persist so long without having been so transformed as to become biologically significant. Adaptation to conditions of night illumination would, however, have no significance worthy of mention for the man of to-day who has replaced natural night illumination by quite different artificial sources of light. The important difference is, therefore, that between sunlight on the one hand and shadow and twilight on the other " (p. 238). We may remark here, in criticism, that civilized man has enjoyed superior artificial illumination for such a short time that it can hardly have exercised any deep-rooted transforming influence upon his sensory functions ; it was only fifty years ago that Edison made his great invention, the development of which has flooded our world with artificial light. Is the vision of men who have as yet no electric lights different from ours ? Can we make owls into diurnal animals by keeping them for a few generations in good illumination ? Is it not true that the difference in illumination between daylight and twilight is more significant, even for civilized man, than the difference between sunlight and shadow ? Members of primitive tribes who were not adapted to deep darkness were lost, and during the war night-blind soldiers found themselves in a very unfortunate position. The contrast between day vision and night vision is phenomeno-logically much more expressive than that between vision in sunlight and in shadow. From a functional point of view, we are reminded of the summation of stimuli in dark adaptation which is manifested generally in binocular vision and as regards magnitude of surface in monocular vision. The dark-adapted eye is predisposed to perceive traces of light, and colour-constancy is sacrificed to this function ; on the other hand, colour-constancy would be endangered if summation of stimuli were not suppressed in binocular vision during light adaptation.

Studies by Achelis and Merkulow [1] likewise indicate that the contrast between daylight vision and twilight vision is more

---

[1] *Zsch. f. Sinnesphysiol.*, 1929, 60.

striking than that between vision in sunlight and in shadow.
Twilight vision is more closely related to affective reactions than
is daylight vision. The light-adapted eye sees movement and
change of position, while the dark-adapted eye sees, rather,
pure movement. Night vision is predominantly subcortical,
daylight vision cortical.

§ 38. The Normal Limits of Vision

For the sake of brevity, we shall call an eye which is
completely adapted to a normally illuminated field a
normally adapted eye. It is important, for our later
discussions, to answer this question : *What is the stimulus
range of the normally adapted eye ?*
What stimulus must act upon a point of the retina
of the normally adapted eye if this point is to be just
distinguishable from the grey field of the closed eyes ?
I fixed a small piece of velvet-black, about 1·5 cm. square,
on a cross of thin black threads stretched before the
opening of a dark tube. In normal illumination the
velvet-black appeared dark grey in front of a lightless
background.
In the following experiments the black was observed
through an episcotister. First we determined the opening
of the episcotister which permitted the square to be just
perceptible to the normally adapted eye. We were
able to decrease the opening to about 2°. This means
that the normally adapted eye is just able to perceive
(as a surface colour) a light-stimulus which has about
$\frac{1 \times 2}{60 \times 360} = \frac{1}{10,800}$ of the light-intensity of an equally
illuminated white paper ; furthermore, the colour is
perceived as a surface colour. This value may be considered as very low. By this method we have determined
the absolute threshold of the normally adapted eye or,
more exactly stated, the differential limen of the normally
adapted eye in terms of the subjective grey.
In calculating the absolute limen of the normally
adapted eye, we have used the light-intensity of our

normally illuminated white paper as the unit of light-intensity. The quotient characterizing this limen would naturally have been lower if we had chosen the intensity of a white paper in direct sunlight as our unit. The illumination produced by direct sunlight is approximately from 60 to 100 times as intense as the illumination of the square in this experiment, the particular ratio depending upon the time of day. We may probably consider the intensity of the white paper, lighted by direct sunlight, as the upper limit of the intensities of the surface colours likely to be seen in nature.

It is of interest to determine here the lowest intensity of the illumination in which *white* objects can still be perceived as approximately *white*. I found it possible to reduce the opening of the episcotister to *less than* 1° and still see through it a white square *on a lightless ground* as " approximately white." [1] With the same opening, a black square on a white ground appears dark grey, *not black*. This shows convincingly how correct Hering was in saying that we cannot obtain deep blacks unless their neighbourhoods have considerable light-intensity.

§ 39. PHENOMENAL CONSTANCY IN OTHER FIELDS

The concept of " constancy," which involves an epistemological problem of the greatest importance, has perhaps its most important root in the psychology of perception. Departing for the moment from the field of colours, we shall show briefly the surprisingly wide range and multiplicity of constancy-phenomena.

Those constancy-phenomena in space-perception which lead to distinctions of real and apparent distance, real and apparent size, and real and apparent form, have always been favourite topics for experimental treatment. I myself have dealt in detail with constancy-phenomena in the field of touch. Since the material is published in my book on touch, I shall not discuss the matter here. I should like to point out, too, that I have also found

---

[1] The white square was, as before, fixed before a dark tube.

interesting constancy-phenomena in the temperature sense.

Werner[1] has demonstrated numerous parallels between sound-constancy and colour-constancy, and v. Hornbostel[2] and Lachmund[3] have given us incidental contributions. Parallels are particularly numerous in the field of hearing, on account of the similarity between visual and auditory perspective.

The constancy-phenomena studied by Fischel[4] in the field of weight perception should also be mentioned. He found it possible to bring his studies into connection with my own investigations of weight estimation by individuals who had undergone Sauerbruch amputations;[5] in these cases I had found that the judgments were strikingly independent of the way in which the weights were lifted.[6] It is indeed astonishing how little the judgment about the magnitude of a weight depends upon which muscles are used in the lifting or upon which particular movements of these muscles are involved. Fischel says, quite rightly, that it is difficult to understand how an empiristic theory could explain his results. Fischel's findings are also interesting in connection with their significance for a theory of comparison. He has shown that no theory of comparison hitherto advanced can do justice to his own experiments. "All these theories are erected on the basis of experiments in which relatively simple impressions were compared with each other." He points out that, under such conditions, the old theories of comparison might have some value, but that another approach is needed in connection with his experiments. He takes as a starting-point Müller's theory of absolute impression. "We assume that when we lift

[1] H. Werner, Grundfragen der Intensitätspsychologie. Leipzig, 1922.

[2] E. v. Hornbostel. Das räumliche Hören. *Handb. d. norm. u. pathol. Physiol.*, 11. Berlin, 1926.

[3] H. Lachmund, *Zsch. f. Psychol.*, 1922, 88.

[4] *Zsch. f. Psychol.*, 1926, 98.

[5] In Sauerbruch amputations individual muscles are attached to separate parts of an artificial limb in such a way as to permit fairly complicated movements of the limb.

[6] D. Katz, *Zur Psychologie des Amputierten und seiner Prothese.* Leipzig, 1921.

a weight, there is established a more or less correct absolute judgment of the objective magnitude of the weight, regardless of what the special bodily apparatus is which is brought into function in the lifting of the weight. . . . Although the objective relationships may be grasped in many ways, the only important condition is that the experience be set off from the purely subjective region in which there can be no immediate comparison, and be transplanted into an objective realm. . . . The views which we have presented hold true for all cases of comparison in which differently organized perceptual contents must be compared from a certain unitary point of view." I agree emphatically with Fischel's account, and may add that the region in which the process of comparison described by Fischel is applicable should be extended to include our experiments with colours. As we have emphasized above, our problem was to establish not identities but equations with reference to certain specific variables. In those cases in which we are aiming at identity, the mode of reaction of the organism may be compared with the operation of scales, where the setting results in an elimination of differences ; but this is not true of the cases represented by our experiments on colour. As yet we have no physical measuring instrument capable of giving us partially equal settings. (Heterochromatic photometry is no exception.) In the light of this consideration, the uniqueness of the phenomena which we have been investigating becomes particularly evident. This short discussion of the process of comparison involved in our experiments will have to be sufficient for present purposes, since we are more concerned with perceptual *contents* than with the functions through which we apprehend them.

§ 40. THE EFFECTS OF CHROMATIC ILLUMINATION

Hering describes the following experiment to illustrate how markedly the chromatic colour of a seen object is independent of the quality of the general illumination.

" I covered one surface of the rectangular prism of a
Bouguer photometer with a flat, non-lustrous brown
paper, and the other with an ultramarine blue paper,
otherwise similar to it. The two papers were carefully
selected for the experiment. I illuminated the brown
paper by means of white daylight reflected from a mirror,
and the other by an ordinary gas-flame or incandescent
lamp. . . . When I looked through the vertical tube of
the photometer, the ' blue ' paper looked exactly like
the ' brown,' if a proper intensity of the artificial light
was used, since in such a light the ' blue ' waves were
completely masked by the ' yellow.' Then I closed the
window-shutters and lighted the entire room with gas-
lamps or incandescent lamps, and removed the two papers
from the apparatus. In spite of the fact that the ' blue '
paper was illuminated by the same artificial light as
before, and was still reflecting the same wave-mixture
into my eyes, it no longer appeared brown, but immediately appeared blue as in daylight, although somewhat
darker. The ' brown ' paper, however, looked brown as
before. It makes no difference in this experiment whether
the observer knows the ' real ' colours of the papers or
not." [1] The fact that the blue paper appears blue even
in lamplight is, according to Hering, a result of chromatic
adaptation of the eye. This theory is inconclusive. The
key to an understanding of this experiment lies in the
recognition of chromatic *illumination* as a phenomenological fact.

If, when our eyes are adapted to neutral light, we
enter a room illuminated by gas or electricity, we notice
a certain tinting of all the colours struck by the artificial
light. This tinting is not equally noticeable in all colours ;
it is stronger in bright colours than in dark colours.
Among the chromatic colours, the oranges undergo the
least change. If we remain in the room for some time the
tinting decreases, at first rapidly, and then more slowly.
It does not become zero, however, even if we remain in
the room for a long time, for some tinting of all the

[1] Hering, VI, p. 15.

colours in the direction of the chromatic illumination persists. The weakening of this tinting depends upon chromatic *adaptation* of the eye. We may now say, in contrast to Hering, that *the tinting of colours in a chromatically illuminated visual field is always lower than it should be, even if we take into full account the chromatic adaptation of the eye at the time.* We are able to prove this statement experimentally.

In these experiments it was convenient to use the principle of the double room, as described by Hering.[1] In a door connecting two rooms (Fig. 9) was an opening O which was so large that an observer, standing in one room, could survey the other when he placed his head in this opening. Room I was lighted by gas. On the wall of this room was a large *white* disc A (standard disc) serving as a test-object. The observer was in room II, which was lighted by daylight ; in this second room a colour-wheel with the comparison disc B was set up close beside O. The observer looked first through the aperture of a

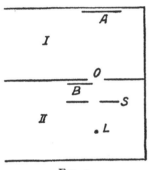

FIG. 9

reduction-screen S which was so arranged that approximately equal parts of the aperture appeared to be filled with portions of the surfaces of A and B. In order to eliminate any differences of hue, brightness or saturation between A and B, we set B (setting I) at 162° yellow and 198° orange. (The colour of A was thus reduced to an illumination normal in quality and intensity.) This value shows immediately what impression the principal disc A would give if it were to emit to the eye, in a normally illuminated room, the same stimulus as under the conditions we have described. Now, when I placed my head in the opening O, the saturation of A became much lower. When I attempted again to make an equation between

[1] *Cf.* Hering, V, p. 522.

A and *B*, by looking at *A* from *O* and at *B* from *L*, I had
to make the following setting (II) on *B* in order to establish
as closely as possible an equation between the colours of
A and *B* : 157° yellow, 47° orange, and 156° white.

By comparing the two settings, we find that disc *A*
appears very much brighter in direct observation than
after reduction. The marked loss in saturation undergone
by *A* cannot be explained in terms of chromatic adaptation
caused by prolonged observation of *A*, since this lasted
only one or two seconds at the most. Although a much
larger part of the visual field was illuminated by chromatic
light in setting II than in setting I, the resulting interaction of retinal elements cannot effect a loss in saturation
of *A of the magnitude here observed*. Let us fasten on a
wall a large sheet of highly saturated coloured paper.
If we approach this paper rapidly so that it appears under
a much greater visual angle than before, we observe no
loss in the saturation of the colour, unless we use further
aids. In this case, the interaction of the retinal points
would be of still greater effect than in the experiment
with chromatic illumination, where only a small part of
the objects filling the visual field reflected chromatic
light of *high* intensity into the eye. Any attempt to
explain the loss in saturation of *A* in terms of a chromatic
adaptation of the eye must appear entirely inadequate as
soon as we examine carefully the situation in which *A*
is seen. Disc *A* is *seen*, not in normal illumination, but
(together with its entire neighbourhood) *in chromatic
illumination*. I emphasize " seen " because this chromatic
illumination is not simply *known* or *inferred*, but is
immediately perceived. The objects, with their colour
qualities, are apprehended as belonging in a *chromatically
illuminated* field. If we neglect this difference in illumination between *A* and *B*, the setting II (as given above)
may also be easily misunderstood. What it means is
this : Of all the possible settings of *B*, this one best
matches in hue and saturation the colour of *A which we
are perceiving in a visual field of reddish-yellow illumination*.
Setting II shows that colour-constancy is no more ideal

in chromatic illumination than in most of the earlier experiments in which achromatic illumination was changed in *intensity*; the colours are tinted, rather, with the colour of the chromatic illumination.

The experiment in which the standard disc A emitted chromatic light which was completely or approximately complementary to the light from the artificial light-source is particularly interesting. The wave-mixture which was reflected by a *blue* standard disc A illuminated by the reddish-yellow light of the gas flame was characterized as follows (setting I) : $B = 330°$ black, $18°$ white, and $12°$ violet. This setting gave the impression of a dark reddish grey, the blue component of the violet being unnoticeable. By the procedure described above we found setting II to be $B = 312°$ black, $16°$ white, and $32°$ violet. In this case, both the blue and the red components were prominent. We have already rejected attempts to explain experiments with chromatic illumination in general in terms of chromatic adaptation, and obviously we shall not adopt this explanation for the particular case in which A has a blue colour. Here, too, the fact is simply that the *genuine* colour (the blue) asserts itself more strongly when the particular quality of its illumination is perceived. It is really no more remarkable that a bluish surface colour should appear in reddish-yellow illumination than that a white should appear in a visual field of reduced illumination or a black in a field of increased illumination. Cases of the latter sort appear less remarkable simply because we are familiar not only with the appearance of white in darkness and of black in light, but also with the intermixture of black and white in the grey colours. We do not encounter such a mixture of blue and yellow (or of red and green) in everyday experience.[1] Since experience has

---

[1] Gelb also found a relative colour-constancy when the colours of an object and of its illumination were complementary. Kaila, *Psychol. Forsch.*, 1923, 3, has questioned this, but I do not consider his doubt justified. Gelb, too, does not accept Kaila's experiments. "These experiments were, in phenomenological respects, performed under very special experimental conditions, and therefore it is questionable whether and to what extent we can draw any general laws from them." Gelb, p. 628.

taught us that in general bright colours are more likely to appear in high and dark colours in low illumination, we have built up a certain relationship between white and strong illumination (light) and between black and weak illumination (darkness). This is also shown in language, for we do not ordinarily distinguish consistently between these different aspects of colour-experience. If there were yellow-blue (or red-green) colours as there are black-whites, we should find less striking the appearance of a blue (or red) colour in yellow (or green) illumination.

It is very difficult to determine exactly the colour of *A* in chromatic illumination. The characterization of blue or greenish-blue surface colours in reddish-yellow illumination is remarkably unstable. If these colours are low in saturation, it may very well happen that observers call the same colour plain grey or yellowish or bluish, even though the stimulation and chromatic adaptation of the eye remain unchanged. We might be justified in speaking here of an indefiniteness of illumination and of an indefiniteness of object colour.

Within a visual field illuminated normally as regards quality we cannot set up colour-impressions which are equal in every respect to those which we see in chromatically illuminated fields. Even Hering overlooked this fact in his experiment described above. In the illumination provided by gas or electricity, we do not see a plain blue (*i.e.*, a blue in illumination of normal quality), but a blue in *reddish-yellow* illumination.

Many light-sources used for illumination (*e.g.*, petroleum light, gas-light, candle-light, certain electric lights) have a pronounced yellow or reddish-yellow tinge. Since even *direct* sunlight causes objects to appear with a reddish-yellow tint, we might expect relative colour-constancy to appear in chromatic illumination only if the special experiences which we have had in reddish-yellow illumination become effective. Experiments with other qualities of illumination do not permit this assumption. I produced a chromatic illumination by enclosing the gas-burner in room I with a sheet of saturated coloured gelatine. When disc *A* was white, as before, we obtained the following three pairs of values, whose meaning should be clear without further explanation :

RED ILLUMINATION

Setting I : $B = 360°$ red.
,,   II : $B = 335°$ red, $25°$ white.

GREEN ILLUMINATION

Setting I : $B = 360°$ green.
,,   II : $B = 323°$ green, $37°$ white.

BLUE ILLUMINATION

Setting I : $B = 360°$ blue.
,,   II : $B = 327°$ blue, $33°$ white.

Chromatic illuminations of the quality and " saturation " of these three are certainly *extremely rare* in everyday life. These experiments are, therefore, of fundamental significance, since they show that relative colour-constancy is possible even under conditions of illumination *with which we have had no previous experience.* This fact shows how little an empiristic theory can do justice to phenomena of colour-constancy.

If we expose green surface colours in red illumination or *vice versa,* we still have the impression of red or green surface colours in complementary illumination, but this impression is not as distinct as in the case of a blue in yellow illumination.

It is possible to perceive a blue surface colour in yellowish illumination *without any trace of a greenish component.* When Brentano [1] states that green is composed of yellow and blue, he is not thinking of an " interpenetration " of these two components as in the cases described above. He is thinking rather of a *normally illuminated* green. According to Brentano, Hering's theory cannot account for the fact that *red-green* colours are not uncommon in painting and in certain technical fields. I must emphasize, on the contrary, that in qualitatively normal illumination I have never encountered surface colours which have shown red and green components as distinctly as certain other colours show, for example, red and blue components.

---

[1] F. Brentano, *Untersuchungen zur Sinnesphysiologie.* Leipzig, 1908.

N

Moderate degrees of saturation of chromatic illumination are best suited to the demonstration of the colour-constancy of seen objects ; if the saturation is too high, the phenomena are less marked. This seems to have been overlooked by some writers who have studied colour-constancy in chromatic illumination. Gelb is thinking of this restriction when he says : " If the chromatic illumination of a disc is too saturated, we get decidedly different results. Colour-constancy may even be entirely lost under such conditions. . . . I have found that both white and chromatic discs show relatively lower colour-constancy as the saturation of the illumination is increased (above a certain point)." [1]

There have been many investigations of the colour-constancy of objects seen in chromatic illumination. One general result of these studies is that colour-constancy is not as pronounced in chromatic illumination as it is in an illumination of abnormal intensity. Bühler was the first to call attention to this fact, although I am inclined to think that he has not done full justice to the real extent of colour-constancy in chromatic illumination. In the studies by Bühler and by his students, as well as by certain other experimenters, we note a tendency to under-estimate colour-constancy in chromatic illumination. This may be due to the fact that they have used experimental procedures which are dominated more or less by physical and physiological purism. They have made their experimental conditions too artificial and have " simplified " them physically and physiologically in such a way that the situations have no biological meaning. Krauss [2] is justified in remarking that " constancy does not exist at all for chromatic colours under conditions of purely monochromatic illumination (which are most unfavourable biologically), and exists only partially even in the case of mixed lights." We must note, however, that colour-constancy is very low even for achromatic illumination if the biological conditions are unfavourable.

[1] Gelb, p. 626.
[2] S. Krauss, *Arch. f. d. ges. Psychol.*, 1928, 62, p. 182.

According to Kardos,[1] we have *a priori* evidence that the colours of objects cannot be seen in monochromatic illumination. This statement is no more admissible than the statement, which might also be made *a priori*, that white can never be perceived in weak illumination.

Gelb explains the lower colour-constancy of objects in chromatic illumination as follows : " The maintenance of the rank-order of achromatically coloured objects as illumination is varied in intensity might be an important factor underlying the severance of illumination and illuminated object ; and this factor does not hold analogously for the chromatic illumination of a visual field composed of achromatic and chromatic colours." [2]

Krauss has made observations of the influence of chromatic illumination upon the impression of depth, and has reached the conclusion that chromatically illuminated spaces are underestimated as regards depth, or manifest a phenomenal shortening. Continued fixation seems to heighten this tendency toward shortening, while a fleeting or impressionistic glance easily leads to a tendency toward overestimation. If we change the intensity of illumination continuously, we observe processes of shrinking and extension of the illuminated spaces.[3]

[1] Bühler-Festschrift, p. 66.   [2] Gelb, p. 678.
[3] Krauss, *op. cit.*, p. 196 ff.

CHAPTER III

How Colours Appear at the Periphery,

§ 41. THE INSISTENCE OF CENTRAL AND
PERIPHERAL COLOURS

LET us stand in front of a uniformly white paper surface
so that as much of the retina as possible is stimulated
by the light reflected from it. Almost the entire visual
field is then filled with white, and we can say with
assurance that *the colour has approximately the same
brightness throughout its extent.* Yet in spite of this
equality in brightness of the central and peripheral parts
of the surface, these differ from each other in a specific
way. The *insistence of the quality white* decreases toward
the peripheral parts, and finally reaches zero, *i.e.*, the
colour vanishes.[1] Thus we see side by side in the visual
field a series of different degrees of insistence of the
same colour. There is a certain relationship between a
colour in reduced illumination and central vision, and
the same colour in normal illumination and peripheral
vision. The two colour-impressions differ, however, in
various respects. Different degrees of *pronouncedness* of
a colour appear only in *different intensities of illumination
of the visual field.* On the other hand, different degrees
of *insistence* of a colour may appear side by side in a visual
field *of uniformly intense illumination.* Indeed, we may
even note such differences in film colours, to which we
cannot ascribe *illumination* in the same sense as to surface
colours. To observe different degrees of insistence of

[1] " I cannot resist the impression that the subjective grey is less insistent
at the periphery than at the centre of the retina. This agrees with Katz's
observation that (even when their brightnesses are the same) white and
grey colours have less insistence at the periphery than at the centre of
the retina." Müller, III, § 2.

a film colour, we may simply look at the uniform colour
of the sky. We might perhaps say that peripheral colours
have less intensity, even though we have rejected this
term in the case of colours presented in low intensity of
illumination.

All the members of the black-white series undergo
changes in insistence in peripheral vision. This is also
true, to a certain extent, of saturated *chromatic* colours.
I cannot agree that the changes in the colours of large
saturated surfaces exposed at the periphery are simply
changes in *saturation*. All the changes in insistence of
colours at the periphery of which we are speaking here
are independent of the particular conditions of illumination of the colours occupying the visual field. Even if a
surface colour is shadowed, it is less insistent at the
periphery than at the centre.

Aubert has shown that a white square exposed peripherally
(at 25° eccentricity) to a light-adapted eye appears only a little
darker than when exposed centrally.[1] He formulates the
hypothesis that " the light-sense shows no important differences
over the entire extent of the retina." Hering states that " one
and the same colour or brightness may penetrate into our
consciousness with different energies, depending upon whether
it is presented centrally or peripherally." [2]

§ 42. COLOUR-CONSTANCY AND PERIPHERAL VISION

Let us fixate monocularly from some distance the centre
of a large grey paper surface set up in a room. The grey
appears in lower degrees of insistence in peripheral parts
of the visual field. If we remove a portion of the grey
paper standing at the side, and replace it by a paper
emitting *just as much* light to the retina but lying farther
or nearer than the grey paper, the impression is not
changed at all. Now let us cut out of the grey paper
surface *F* a portion lying toward one side, and place at

---

[1] Aubert, *Physiologie der Netzhaut.* Breslau, 1864, p. 92 ff.
[2] Hering, VI, p. 108.

some distance behind it a paper surface *a* of the same retinal effect as the grey paper (*i.e.*, of higher albedo), or hang by means of fine threads *in front of* lateral portions of the grey surface a piece of achromatic paper *b*, again of the same retinal effect as F (*i.e.*, of lower albedo). In neither case do we note a change in the situation. Thus we have three papers, of different brightnesses and different intensities of illumination, judged as equally bright (and equally illuminated) when they are seen with the retinal periphery, and judged as different in brightness and in intensity of illumination when they are seen with

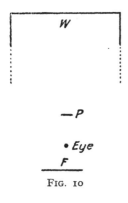

FIG. 10

central parts of the retina. If *a* and *b* are of higher or lower intensity than the grey surface F, they are judged to be as bright as a portion of F which is equal to them in intensity. From these observations we may draw the following conclusion : If peripherally perceived colours are not localized in such a way as to appear in an illumination different from that seen at the centre, our impression of them is determined by the kind of illumination perceived at the centre of the retina.

If the situation permits us to realize that the objects seen peripherally lie in an illumination different from that at the centre, the impressions of these objects are determined essentially by the conditions of their own illumination ; at the same time, the central objects present the colour characteristics which correspond to their own illumination. We may easily convince ourselves of this in the following way (Fig. 10). A small piece of paper P of any colour is hung near a window F. This paper appears in the prevailing illumination. Now let us fixate monocularly a point (real or imaginary) upon the wall W of the room lying behind the paper. Then in spite of the fact that the colours of the remote wall and of the objects in its neighbourhood are projected on peripheral parts of the retina, they are judged to be about the same as if the more brightly illuminated paper in front of them did not lie in the visual field. It is the much weaker illumination of the wall behind which is perceived, apparently because it now occupies most of the visual field.

Two pieces of cardboard (about 7 cm. square) were fastened at right angles to each other ; one of them was covered with white and the other with dark grey paper. They were placed by a window in such a way that the dark grey surface g was normally illuminated and the white surface w was in shadow ; the latter, however, after it had been reduced to the illumination of g, appeared somewhat darker than g—a fact which makes the significance of the observations to be described even clearer. The observer sat about 50 cm. in front of the cardboard surfaces so that they formed approximately the same angles with the median plane of his head. The centre of the line in which the surfaces intersected was at the height of his eyes. At the angle of intersection of the surfaces we placed a straight wire, which projected equally beyond the top and bottom edges of the cardboards, and stood out clearly from the neutral background H. When the observer fixated monocularly a point in the line of intersection of the surfaces, the *shadowed* cardboard appeared much brighter ; but when he fixated the upper or lower portion of the wire, the colour-impression changed. If the fixation point was moved so far up or so far down that both coloured surfaces were projected upon peripheral parts of the retina (at about 30° eccentricity), the observer no longer noted any difference between the illuminations of the two surfaces. Furthermore, the surface w, which had appeared brighter in central vision, now appeared darker. It was not easy to make reports about the illuminations in which the two surfaces g and w seemed to lie. The observers were most inclined to say that they lay in the same illumination as that prevailing at the fixation point. The two surfaces had lost their previous orientation toward the observer, but it was impossible to say with any certainty whether or not they lay in the *same* plane. Then we placed two fixation points upon the wire, one some distance toward the top and the other the same distance toward the bottom, and compared the colours obtained by fixating the two in turn. The impression of different illuminations of the coloured surfaces disappeared *sooner*, and at the same time the surface *w* darkened *more quickly*, when the eye was moved downward. Equally eccentric points of the upper and lower halves of the retina thus behave differently as regards the perception of colours lying in different illuminations. *The upper half of the retina is more efficient than the lower in apprehending conditions of illumination.* I was unable to discover any analogous differences between temporal and nasal portions of the retinal periphery. I carried out incidental experiments in which the coloured surface *w* was normally illuminated, surface *g* was lighted by direct sunlight, and the two colours were approximately equal after reduction. In peripheral vision, the impression of the difference in illumination between the two coloured surfaces again vanished, and they appeared about equally bright. We may also make similar observations by lighting the two surfaces *g* and *w* with artificial illuminations of different intensities.

How can these observations be explained? There is a difference between central and peripheral parts of the retina in the apprehension of spatial relationships. In monocular peripheral vision, the localization of a surface as regards depth becomes much less definite than in central vision. Our uncertainty becomes still greater when we are asked to judge the *orientation* of a peripherally perceived surface in relation to ourselves or to the light-sources. It is only under certain particular conditions that impressions are localized as regards distance and oriented with respect to the observer as definitely as are those seen centrally. If I look with one eye at a uniform surface occupying the entire visual field, the localization and orientation of the peripheral parts of the surface are never as definite as those of the central parts ; but if I apprehend the totality in front of me as a unitary surface, I can make an *approximately* correct judgment about the localization and orientation of the peripheral portions. If the factors permitting us to apprehend the totality as *one* surface are ruled out, we have unfavourable conditions for judging with assurance the localization and orientation of the peripheral parts of the surface. Now, if it is true that I cannot correctly orient a coloured surface, the basis for the normal constitution of the impression of illumination is also lacking. In our experiments a perfectly adequate localization and orientation of the two coloured surfaces w and g cannot be formed in terms of centrally projected objects. The centrally perceived wire to which the fixation point is attached does, of course, form with the two surfaces a unitary configuration causing them to be localized at about the same distance ; but this does not make their mutual orientation clear. The background H, which is visible centrally, together with the wire, is even less adequate as a basis for a judgment concerning the mutual orientation of surfaces w and g. The consequence is that the two surfaces are only indefinitely localized ; we do not recognize the difference in the orientation of the two surfaces. Under these conditions the colours are referred to a common plane, and hence are seen approximately in their reduction values.

Another aspect of our results may be explained in the following way : The retinal periphery is unable to perceive microstructure distinctly, because the rods are incapable of this function. According to our earlier discussions, the perception of microstructure provides the basis for the judgment of the material of an object. This fact renders possible a convincing demonstration of the inferiority of the retinal periphery upon which we have touched. By means of a rod, let us introduce into the visual field from the side, and about 50 cm. from the eye, small pieces of different materials (wood, coal, cloth, paper, metal, etc.), whose forms and colours permit no inferences about their material composition. It is best to use objects of the same form and colour. The material which is recognized without any difficulty in foveal vision is quite puzzling in peripheral vision. Indeed, it is actually astounding to find how small that region of the visual field is which permits us to apprehend the material of an object simply through the peculiarity of its surface structure. Hence, if we are observing peripherally the two coloured surfaces w and g, we should not perceive the difference in the distinctness of their surface structure which is conditioned by the physical difference in illumination. Observation confirms this hypothesis. We no longer apprehend differences in structure. The consequence is that in so far as the perception of the difference in surface structure between g and w is an aid in apprehending centrally the illuminations of these two surfaces, this aid must be lacking in peripheral vision. According to what we have said, the difference in brightness between g and w should be the same in extremely eccentric vision as it is after reduction to the same illumination. This is actually the case. From these observations we may draw the following conclusion : *To the extent to which differences in the localization of colours and in the distinctness of their surface structure recede in peripheral vision, the apprehension of differences in their illumination also becomes more difficult, and to the same extent the colours themselves come to be determined directly by the intensities of the corresponding stimuli.*

Lights and shadows lying upon an object pass through very fine gradations into normally illuminated colours. As we have shown above in connection with one of Hering's experiments, these delicate transitions in brightness are not unimportant in giving rise to impressions of superimposed shadow or, we may add, of superimposed light. It is only within a very small region (perhaps limited to the fovea) that the retina is able to distinguish these fine gradations in brightness. Hence lights and shadows which fall upon small areas of the visual field cannot be perceived as such with peripheral parts of the retina, even though they may lie only a little to one side of the point of clearest vision. Even if the eccentricity is very slight, a spot of shadow or light is seen as a modification of a local colour.

§ 43. MODES OF APPEARANCE AT THE PERIPHERY

What is the mode of appearance of peripherally perceived colour ? When we are perceiving an object that extends over both central and peripheral parts of the retina, we cannot deny that even its peripheral parts have the character of surface colour, even though a transition to *film colour* may be noted. A colour which would be apprehended in central vision as a film colour can be apprehended peripherally even as a surface colour if proper central determinants are present. This is illustrated by the following observation. The observer fixated a point in a large paper surface *P*. A peripheral portion of the paper was removed, and a paper of the same retinal effect was placed behind this opening *O*. The situation could be arranged in such a way that the colour of the paper seen *directly* through the opening *O* appeared as a film colour. The colour of the paper no longer had this mode of appearance in peripheral vision. There could be no doubt that it looked very much more like a surface colour. It was impossible to say positively that it appeared distinctly as a surface colour ; it might be better to say that *the entire paper P exhibited essentially the appearance of surface colour*, no part of it standing out in any different mode of appearance. If an object which would appear as a surface in direct vision is exposed peripherally, and there are no central determinants which might cause it to appear as a surface, then the colour at the periphery either resembles or actually appears as a film colour. Now let us look at a large uniform surface and, by means of a thin rod, introduce an object (such as a paper) into the visual field from the periphery. The object is seen at the periphery as film colour, and this impression persists until the object appears almost at the centre.

The experiments described in this section demonstrate the important fact that we must ascribe to the centre of the retina, in addition to its generally recognized superiority in spatial perception, other functions which have hitherto been scarcely considered. *The centre of the retina, and it alone, makes possible the perception of pronounced surface colours.* Since, as we have shown, shadowing and lighting appear only in connection with surface colours, we should be able to perceive shadowing and lighting distinctly only with the centre of the retina. Observations described in preceding sections confirm this satisfactorily.

Gelb's observations of the return in his patients of surface colour perception which they had lost agree very closely with my views about the significance of the centre of the retina for the perception of surface colours. Surface colours first began to return in central vision, within a visual angle of about 3°, while the parts seen more peripherally still had the character of film colour. Wherever the patient looked, the colour seemed to adhere more closely to the paper. "Our discovery that perception of surface colours returned first at the fovea may serve as a striking confirmation of Katz's view that it is primarily the fovea which has the function of mediating the perception of clear-cut surface colour." [1]

If we wish to examine objects quite closely, we usually look at them with the centre of the fovea, or inspect them from all sides. We do this because the centre of the retina is superior in visual acuity. Memorial impressions of the forms of seen objects are thus based normally only upon the activity of the relatively central parts of the retina. According to general laws of practice, it seems at least plausible that the centre of the retina or the corresponding neural apparatus should acquire, in addition to its innate (histologically determined) superiority, a functional superiority in apprehending the forms of

[1] Gelb, p. 651.

objects. Just as the perception of the forms of seen objects involves relatively central parts of the retina, their recognition will likewise originate primarily from such points. Now if objects in general are recognized most easily at the centre of the retina, this should hold specifically for objects to which we ascribe memory colours. *We may assume, accordingly, that the memory colour of an object is generally aroused most easily when the centre of the retina is activated.*

The different histological structures of the centre and periphery of the retina contribute to the functional differentiation of the two corresponding neural centres as regards colour-constancy. Perhaps a differentiation of the nervous centres connected with different parts of the retina may also explain the different capacities of the upper and lower parts of the retina,[1] a difference which can hardly be explained entirely in terms of the superior acuity of the upper part of the retina. Since most events occur " below " rather than " in front of," and only rarely " above," our eyes, the upper parts of the retina, which are thus more frequently used, become better adapted to their tasks.

In those amnesias which involve familiarity of objects, the influence of memory colour may recede while colour-constancy, in so far as it depends upon a histologically determined superiority of the centre of the retina, remains normal. There appears to have been a loss of memory colours in a case of cortical blindness described by E. Wehrli.[2] " His (the patient's) memory for the form and appearance of familiar objects was markedly disturbed. Moreover, he showed complete amnestic colour-blindness ; in imagination all objects (grass, blood, etc.) appeared to him as black."

As we have seen, the memory colour of an object is aroused most easily by processes at the centre of the retina, but if an object of very characteristic form has been projected upon peripheral points of the retina, it is possible for its memory colour to be reproduced from that region.

[1] *Cf.* p. 200.
[2] *Arch. f. Ophthalm.*, 1906, 62, p. 288.

I cut a semicircular piece *a* (Fig. 11), about 8 cm. in diameter, from a piece of cardboard covered with black paper. On the area *b* which, together with area *a*, made up a complete circle *V*, I pasted a coloured paper. On the side of the cardboard turned away from the observer I pasted over *a* such a combination of coloured gelatine films that, when a piece of white paper at a suitable distance behind *a* was illuminated appropriately, *a* appeared to an observer looking at the field from the front as equal to *b* in hue, saturation and brightness. When the observer examined these colour-areas *a* and *b* from a distance of 15–20 cm., first moving his eyes over points of *a* and then over points of *b*, he had the distinct impression that the upper area *a* represented a *transparent*

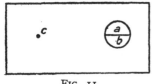

FIG. 11

coherence plane and the lower a surface colour. The surface colour perceived behind the transparent area appeared in chromatic illumination. When the observer fixated central parts of the coloured fields *a* and *b*, their extreme parts were projected upon the periphery of the retina. Yet the entire extent of the area *a*, and not merely the parts whose images fell upon the centre of the retina, appeared transparent. This observation confirms our generalization[1] that the retinal periphery may mediate a colour-impression of the same mode of appearance as that at the centre of the retina if certain determinants lead to an assimilation of the modes of appearance of the centrally and peripherally perceived colours.[2] Now we eliminated the effect of such determinants in the following way. From a distance of about 30 cm. the observer fixated monocularly a point *c* on the cardboard lying about 12 cm. from the centre of the circle *V*,

---

[1] *Cf.* p. 203.
[2] "The determinants originating from the centre consist of configural relationships" (Fuchs, II, p. 312). Gelb follows Fuchs's view. "Under such conditions, certain assimilations following the laws of configuration apply. This has nothing to do with the effects of past experience. . . ." (Gelb, p. 642).

so that the two semicircles *a* and *b* were projected upon peripheral parts of the retina. The mode of appearance of *a* was no longer different from that of *b*, and the two semicircular fields fused into a unitary circle. It was not easy to describe the real mode of appearance of the circular field of colour. It did not, in any case, give an impression of transparency. The directly inspected part of the black cardboard, and the parts of it which were seen indirectly, appeared as *surface colours*. Now the appearance of the circle as film colour may perhaps be attributed to the fact that the great difference in brightness between the black and the colour of the circle did not favour an apprehension of the two as colours of the *same* mode of appearance (in this case, as surface colours). Our experiment shows that the impression of transparent colour may not be had with peripheral parts of the retina unless apprehension as a transparent colour is determined from the centre of the retina. It is noteworthy that the transparence of colours disappears at distances at which surface colours can still be perceived, even when no determinants from the centre are effective.

Distinct *volume colours* are unobservable at the periphery. Unless a voluminous mode of appearance is aroused by processes at the centre of the retina, what we see is film colour. *Lustre* disappears completely in extreme peripheral vision. Objects (such as metal objects) which seem to have great lustre in central vision appear in peripheral vision to be luminous, especially if the intensity of illumination of the rest of the visual field is lower. Under these conditions, objects of polished copper show a luminosity of surprising beauty. Lustre which has vanished in peripheral vision may return if the object at the periphery is moved ; but in such a case the lustre is never as distinct as in central vision.

The impression of *luminosity* persists at the periphery, although it never has a distinctly voluminous character. The impression of luminosity is present at the periphery only if strong lights are used. When transparent colours

are moved to the periphery, they lose their character
sooner than do surface colours. The impressions of
voluminousness and lustre likewise disappear sooner than
do surface colours. The differentiation in this respect
between parts of the retina of different eccentricities
seems to be of some significance for the theory of the
modes of appearance of colour.

We might expect that an eye completely deprived of
peripheral vision might suffer no loss, since the centre
of the retina is able to mediate colours of any mode of
appearance. All that we have demonstrated, however,
is that the retinal periphery in isolation is inferior to the
centre. The question whether the centre of the retina
would retain its full efficiency without the co-operation
of the periphery is still unanswered. We can exclude
peripheral vision artificially, as Purkinje did, by means
of small tubes. Let us hold to our eye the end of a short
tube, which is covered at the other end by a piece of
cardboard with a small opening, providing a visual field
of only a few degrees. Since the perceived sector of the
external world must not be too large, the coloured objects
for judgment should be exposed at a short distance from
the hole in the cardboard. It is best to use a tube of
milk-glass. By wrapping this with various layers of tissue-
paper, we can supply approximately the same amount of
light to all parts of the retina, and can form contrast
relationships such as exist when the tube is removed.
Except for the small central area, the visual field is filled
with a colour appearing as a film colour. When we
exclude the periphery of the retina, a change appears
in the colours lying in the central field of vision. If we
are to see surface colours in this small visual area, we must
fulfil the same conditions as if peripheral vision were not
excluded. If we fill the visual field with objects which
are individually unfamiliar, we no longer apprehend the
nature of the conditions of illumination with as much
assurance as if vision were completely unimpeded. The
conditions are relatively most favourable if the objects
are *normally* illuminated. Our impression of them is not

essentially different from what it is in an unlimited visual field. On the other hand, the colour-impressions of objects in illumination of abnormal intensity or quality are likely to be changed, since it is impossible to give with assurance any reports about the nature of their illumination. (This is true for the stationary eye. If the eye moves, it is possible to a certain extent, through successive perception of the parts of the visual field, to survey more adequately the conditions of illumination.) The illumination creates a strange impression. If we are looking at objects in an unrestricted visual field, it is always possible to make judgments about the prevailing illumination, but such judgments are much more difficult in the small visual field. With a marked change of illumination it is even impossible to report with any certainty whether or not the illumination or the colour of the objects has changed.

These experiments with the tube show that *the periphery contributes to a large extent to the constitution of the impression of the quality and intensity of the illumination prevailing in the visual field*. If peripheral vision is excluded, we become very uncertain about the intensity and quality of the illumination prevailing in the central field of vision. In mediating the impression of clear-cut surface colours, the centre of the retina is independent of the periphery, but a correct perception of the illumination prevailing in the visual field is impossible in central vision without the aid of the periphery.

It is striking with what assurance the colours of normally illuminated objects are perceived, even in a very small central visual field, if their surface structures are quite distinct. This fact reveals a remarkably accurate absolute memory for all colour-qualities—a capacity which is closely related to the perception of clear surface structure. If we eliminate the perception of surface structure by using a lens whose effect cannot be counteracted by accommodation, we can no longer apprehend with any certainty the attributes of colours lying in the small central visual field.

o

It is quite probable that in severe pathological narrowing of the field of vision, the disturbance of orientation
in otherwise familiar space is determined, in part, by the
patients' inability to survey the conditions of illumination.
Here I should like to call attention to certain laws of
colour-vision which have been considered less in the
pathology of vision than in the psychology of normal
vision.   If isolated parts of the retinal periphery lack
colour-constancy, and if, on the other hand, the centre
of the retina reaches its full efficiency in this respect only
through co-operation with the periphery, we cannot
dismiss the idea that, under normal conditions, *the sphere
representing the projection-field of all retinal elements must
always be conceived, so far as colour-constancy is concerned,
as a functional totality.*   If it is true that impressions of
lustre, volume and transparency can be aroused distinctly
only by processes at the centre of the retina, and if the
phenomena of colour-constancy are distinct only in that
region, v. Monakow's theory concerning the rôle of the
macula is given further support.   "The function of the
macula is more than that of perceiving light as extended,
for the macula plays a further rôle in utilizing all the
details in the visual field for the formation of light-
sensations. . . ."[1]

> We usually turn the macula toward objects which are arousing
> our attention through a non-visual sense, *e.g.*, contact.   It is
> probable, therefore, that the neural loci connected with the
> macula assume, in the course of experience, a more intimate
> and more complex interconnection with other spheres, *e.g.*,
> that of touch, than do those corresponding to peripheral parts
> of the retina.   This alone should make it clear why the macula
> is better insured against injurious influences.

Just as peripheral vision may be disturbed in one way
or another, macular vision may be injured to various
extents by a central scotoma.   Since we ascribe to the
macula very particular functions in perceiving the various
modes of appearance of colour, these modes of appearance

[1] *Ergebn. d. Physiol.*, 1902, I, 2, p. 661.

should be disturbed when central vision is eliminated or injured. In so far as the functioning of the centre of the retina, when colour-constancy phenomena are present, involves an individual adjustment (in the biological sense), every other part of the retina must be capable of a similar adjustment. We should expect this, for example, in the cases of " vicarious maculæ "[1] in individuals who squint.

§ 44. Some Theoretical Considerations

There is an hypothesis that the retinal periphery has a primordial type of vision, or represents relatively early stages in the development of vision. We sometimes find this hypothesis including the further assumption that we can still follow, in individual life, the progress from that original vision to the present type of vision. Here we find represented either the view that the transition takes place by way of learning or personal experience, or the view that learning or experience is unimportant, and that new structures of colour-perception are brought into being by inner maturation. In the one case the development would be continuous, in the other case saltatory.[2] We shall not express here any opinion about the basic hypothesis, but shall simply bring together, from the facts of this chapter, what seems relevant to that " primordial " type of vision.

The slightest displacement from the centre of the retina causes the impression that lights and shadows are lying upon surface colours to disappear. The perception of such superimposed lights and shadows should accordingly belong among the most recent achievements of the neural organs. Transparent film colours, distinct. volume colours and lustre are *not* perceptible in peripheral vision. According to our earlier analyses, the first two of these modes of appearance and the last are usually

[1] *Cf., e.g.*, A. Bielschowsky, *Arch. f. Ophthalm.*, 1900, 50.
[2] The necessity for our making greater allowance for saltatory tendencies in development has been emphasized by D. and R. Katz, *Gespräche mit Kindern.* Berlin, 1928, p. 24 ff.

presented in connection with surface colours. If the latter are lacking, these three modes of appearance cannot be seen distinctly. Since, according to our observations, there are no clear-cut surface colours at the periphery, these too would seem to be late developments. Yet since they may be perceived at greater eccentricities than transparent colours, volume colours and lustre, they seem to belong to an earlier level in the development of colour-perception than do these three. It is particularly interesting that filmy *luminosity* is, from our point of view, as " old " as the film colours, since it may be observed distinctly at the periphery. According to our earlier analyses, luminous film colours are distinguished from non-luminous film colours only by their greater brightness, if we disregard the tendency toward voluminousness which they sometimes show. Strongly lustrous objects might also have appeared first as luminous, since they give us the impression of luminosity at the periphery.

Speculation concerning the primordial vision of the retinal periphery might be extended to include perception of size, form and movement. I have given some consideration to the primordial perception of movement in my book on touch.

PART IV

TRANSPARENT AND TRANSLUCENT COLOURS

§ 45. SPATIAL COMBINATIONS OF CHROMATIC AND ACHROMATIC COLOURS

OBSERVATIONS of colours appearing through other colours have occasionally been made in connection with hypnosis,[1] and in pathology in those cases of visual hallucination in which objects lying behind the hallucinatory image are seen through it. Quantitative experiments with transparent and translucent colours, chromatic as well as achromatic, are of considerable interest in connection with the analyses to which we have subjected these phenomena.

First let us carry out an imaginary experiment. Let us bring before our eyes a light-emitting episcotister, large enough to fill the whole visual field and without any visible structure which betrays its presence. The objects lying behind the episcotister will now appear in a visual field, the intensity of whose illumination will be reduced according to the size of the episcotister opening, and at the same time the colours of all the objects will tend toward a *brightness equality* in keeping with the intensity of the light emitted by the episcotister. This effect will vary directly with the intensity of the light coming from the episcostister, with the result that the visual field will in general appear either *more intensely* or *less intensely lighted* with the episcotister than without it; never, however, is the tendency toward equalization of intensity absent. This equalization must impair the perception of objects. The finest details in the surface

---

[1] The first experiments in this field are reported in R. Heidenhain, *Der sogenannte tierische Magnetismus*. Breslau, 1880. Further references are to be found in the article by Levy-Suhl (*cf.* § 53).

structures of the objects are first to suffer from the superposition of light, whereas the vividly contrasting boundaries of objects withstand it most successfully.[1] It is the reduction in clearness of contour or of surface structure of objects, under conditions of lighting which would never, or at any rate never to the same extent, result in such a reduction, which produces the impression that the objects are being partially obscured by an overlay of volume colour, and distinguishes it from the normal impression. This imaginary experiment was realized, not by means of an epicostister, but in another way. I made use of a glass vessel, shaped in the form of one of the rectangular cooling tanks frequently employed for projection purposes. This vessel could be filled with variously coloured fluids. If the fluid used was water, to which a small quantity of milk had been added, one had the impression, when viewing the landscape through it, that one was looking at objects through a space filled with a whitish mist. By a variation of the quantity of milk in the water, it was possible to effect artificial variations of the thickness of the mist. Although the fluid layer was only moderately thick (about ⅓ cm.), one had the impression that the mist was extended through the whole of space. When observation was binocular the spatiality of the mist was clearer, and at the same time the objects seen through it stood out more clearly as to contour and genuine colour. With this arrangement it is not difficult to verify the observation already made that mist remains visible only as long as *objects* can be seen through it ; the mist disappears as soon as this condition ceases to be fulfilled, *e.g.*, in the case of the sky. The use of a milk solution in the vessel resulted in general in a heightening of brightness throughout the visual field. If this is replaced by water, to which black dye has been added,

---

[1] In this connection one striking application of the principle of the episcotister to the determination of the brightness of chromatic colours deserves mention. Matthaei considers the brightness of the colours of two episcotisters—one chromatic, the other achromatic—to be equal if it is possible " to look through each of them at a test object containing a variety of achromatic steps, and recognize the same number in each case." R. Matthaei, *Zsch. f. Sinnesphysiol.*, 1928, 59, p. 271.

the visual field undergoes a reduction in brightness, analogous to that produced by a smoked glass. Dye solutions and smoked glass have the effect of reducing illumination, without at the same time superimposing a uniform light on the visual field. If, however, a little milk is added to the dye solution, the impression of a grey or blackish mist is produced. If *clear chromatic* solutions are used instead of the achromatic solutions, the objects seen through them appear suffused with chromatic light, like objects seen through coloured glasses. If a little milk is added to these clear chromatic solutions, the space then appears as filled with a *coloured mist*. In this way quite remarkable colour-impressions can be produced, impressions which one seldom if ever encounters in nature.

§ 46. THE LAWS OF FIELD SIZE

To the wall of a brightly tinted room are attached a printed sheet, a thermometer and a few other relatively small objects. The differences in brightness between these objects and the other parts of the wall included in the visual field are quite small. One is justified in assuming, consequently, that, if an observer regards this wall from varying distances, the quantities of light affecting his eye will be sufficiently *constant* to meet the requirements of the experiments to be described. A smoked glass with a transmission factor of about 1/30 is fastened in a frame, large enough to include a free area of about 5 sq. cm. of the glass. Perpendicular to the glass surface is attached a cardboard projection, 30 cm. long, the free end of which is placed against the bridge of the nose, so that the distance between glass and eye may be held constant. The margin of the frame is about 1 cm. wide, and beyond it one can see the objects filling out the rest of the visual field. The smoked glass must be held in such a way that no disturbing light-reflexes are produced in the eye which is nearer the light-source.[1] The observer first places himself as close as

[1] A black cloth mask is recommended for such observations.

possible to the printed sheet (which he observes mono-cularly through the smoked glass) without permitting shadows from his head and the glass itself to be cast on the surface. In my observations the minimum distance between the glass and the paper was about 10 cm. The paper is normally illuminated, but those parts which are seen through the smoked glass naturally undergo a con-siderable darkening because of the absorption of light by the smoked glass. While they appear to be illuminated about as strongly as the rest of the visual field, their brightness is perceived as reduced in direct proportion to the reduction in transmitted light effected by the smoked glass. Now let the observer step some distance back from the wall, without changing his fixation, so that not only the printed sheet but also a large section of the wall, with the objects attached to it, can be seen through the smoked glass. The size of the retinal area affected by light coming through the smoked glass will remain approximately constant for all positions of the observer, and consequently the total amount of light affecting the retina will remain approximately the same. Consequently no brightness change in the sheet of paper, resulting from the observer's change of position, can be referred to simultaneous brightness contrast. Any changes in colour observed in the central part of that section of the visual field observed through the smoked glass are, then, clearly not to be reduced to changes in conditions of retinal excitation.[1] Nevertheless, these changes are actually very marked. As the observer steps away from the printed sheet, there develops the impression that *the intensity of illumination both within and without the smoked glass area is changing; within this area there is a perceptible reduction in illumination.* This impression becomes steadily clearer the farther the observer steps back, *i.e.*, *the larger the section of the external world visible through the smoked glass.* Within the area in which the illumination appears reduced, the colours of objects undergo those

---

[1] It is assumed here that simultaneous contrast is dependent primarily upon peripheral conditions.

changes which our previous experiments with reduced illuminations would lead us to expect. In order to obtain greater distances, I repeated these observations in the open air. As object for observation I selected the wall of a house, painted fairly uniformly and containing a few windows. I walked away from the house until finally the whole wall was visible through the glass. The wall then appeared clearly as though it were in natural twilight. A whole row of houses, seen in the same way, produced the same impression. It is important to note that the reduced illumination, seen in the smoked-glass area, and the normal illumination, seen in the rest of the visual field, merge *immediately* into each other.

We rejected the suggestion that the changes in colour-impression, observed in the visual area seen through the smoked glass, could be explained in terms of retinal excitation. Quite apart from the size of the observed changes, their qualitative character alone would convince us that they *cannot* be referred to such peripheral factors. Simultaneous contrast might possibly account for a change in *brightness*, but it could never account for the change in *illumination* observed in these experiments.

Let us summarize our observations briefly. If within an area of the visual field which is filled with objects the intensity of the illumination is uniformly reduced, the changed impression thus induced varies with the way in which this area is filled. If only a small section of the external world is seen within it, the colours of the objects are then in essential correspondence with the intensity of retinal excitation and with the illumination perceived in the total visual field. If a large section of the external world is seen within this area (at a correspondingly greater distance), the illumination within it appears reduced, and the colours undergo such changes as they would undergo if the illumination of the whole visual field were reduced.

One would naturally expect corresponding effects where the illumination of a section of the visual field was increased instead of decreased. And this is, in fact, the case. It can be demonstrated in the following way. Direct sunlight falls upon part of the visual field, and observation is made through a hole in a cardboard screen, held in such a way that it is normally illuminated and always at the same distance from the eye. Viewed from a great distance the sunlit part of the visual field looks intensely illuminated, whereas when viewed from close at hand its illumination seems normal. The surface colours, of course, undergo changes in keeping with the changes in illumination.

One might expect, too, *that impressions of changing illumination within a visual area presented through a smoked glass would increase in clarity with increases in the size of the smoked glass.* We can convince ourselves of this fact by standing at some distance from the wall of a room and varying the position of a smoked glass between the wall and our eyes. When the glass is far from the eye, the brightness of what lies behind it is directly in keeping with the amount of light passing through the glass and the general illumination of the room. The greatest change in the impression is found when the smoked glass is held so close to the eye that the whole visual field appears in reduced illumination. The changes in retinal process brought about here by changes in the position of the glass are obviously greater than in the previous experiment. Nevertheless they are quite incapable of accounting for the phenomena observed, because here, too, we are dealing not merely with *brightness* changes but also with changes in *illumination* impression.

The smoked glass may be replaced by a *chromatically coloured* glass, and analogous results are obtained. If we hold a coloured glass of medium size immediately in front of the objects we are observing, that part of the visual field which is seen through the glass appears as definitely coloured, and the saturation of the colours corresponds to the saturation the same reflected light would produce in a correspondingly illuminated field. If now we look at a larger section of our surroundings through the glass, or simply take a larger glass, the objects cease to appear merely as coloured and are seen instead as *chromatically illuminated* ; and at the same time the objects appear more or less in their natural colours. This consistent relationship between change in illumination impression of part of the visual field and change in its *real* size (*i.e.*, change in retinal size) or in *apparent* size (retinal size held constant) may be expressed in the form of two laws. These we may term the *first and second laws of field size.*[1]

It is clear from the derivation of the laws of field size that the visual field must present a certain articulation if the phenomena described are to be easily observable. If the visual field is less articulated, or is uniformly filled with a single surface colour, they are less clear. And it might be mentioned, although the fact is obvious, that they disappear completely when film colours are substituted for surface colours. Finally, it is worth noting that anything which serves to enhance the phenomena of colour-constancy tends also to strengthen phenomena which underlie the laws of field size.

§ 47. PROJECTED AFTER-IMAGES

A negative after-image projected on a surface has the same effect on the objects seen through it as though it were a transparent or translucent medium. The colours are not simply tinted with the colour of the after-image, but one has rather the impression of a *change in illumination* within the area occupied by the after-image. Surface colours are, it is true, tinted with the colour of the after-image, and the degree of this tinting follows the laws of field size. The validity of the second of these laws may be tested in the following way. Project a small, strong after-image on a wall, which has a number of objects attached to it, as in the case described on p. 215. When the after-image has developed clearly, step away from the wall without changing your fixation in the least. With an increase in the distance from the wall you will

[1] The way in which an increase in the real or apparent size of a part of the visual field affects the perception of illumination is similar to the way in which attention is related to the real and apparent size of spatial structures ; *cf.* E. R. Jaensch, *Zentralblatt f. Physiol.*, 1910, 24, p. 94 ff.

find that its genuine colours become steadily more pronounced. At the same time, as the after-image becomes larger it will lose in clearness and you will have instead the impression of a different illumination within the area covered by the after-image. These changes in impression cannot be due to the recession of the after-image with elapsing time, for they are equally clear when the procedure is reversed. When you approach the wall without changing your fixation-point, the after-image simply becomes clearer and stronger, and the impression of a deviating illumination disappears. Those who find it difficult to move without shifting fixation can obtain the same result by producing the same after-image several times at different distances from the wall.

The validity of the first law of field size is also easy to demonstrate by means of negative after-images. The after-effects of a chromatic adaptation which extends over the whole retina are easily apprehended as changes in illumination, and for this reason are scarcely noticeable.

§ 48. Mirrored Colours

The pictures seen reflected in a piece of plain ground glass are sometimes difficult to observe, if at the same time a good deal of light is coming directly through the glass from objects behind. Mirror-images are quite clear, however, if the back of the glass is painted black, preferably with varnish. Only part of the light falling directly on such a glass is reflected, and this reduction in the reflected light is uniform for the whole surface. It follows then that, as long as the amount of diffuse reflection is small, objects seen in a black mirror ought to look somewhat the same as objects seen through a lightless or almost completely lightless episcotister. And this is, in fact, the case. Objects seen in a dark mirror are seen as in reduced illumination, and their colours present a correspondingly changed appearance. At the same time their contours and surface structure are scarcely less clear than they are when seen through an episcotister transmitting the same amount of light. Both laws of field size hold true for the impression of reduced illumination produced by mirroring.

The results of mirroring surfaces in coloured mirrors can be readily predicted from the foregoing. Such mirrors can be easily produced with coloured paint. The amount of chromatic light reflected can be controlled by a variation of the position of the mirror with reference to the light-source, and this is reflected evenly by the whole surface. Thus the conditions of retinal stimulation are approximately the same as if objects were seen through a coloured fluid that is not quite clear. The impression created is exactly the same as if the reflected objects were seen through a coloured mist, and the surface colours are changed in almost exactly the same way as if a coloured episcotister had been used. It is almost unnecessary to say that here, too, the phenomena follow the two laws of field size.

§ 49. A Critique of the Doctrine of Unity

Observations such as the foregoing are reported, as a matter of fact, by Helmholtz. He used polished mahogany plates for mirrors, and interpreted the resulting severance of the impression into colour of reflecting surface and, behind it, colour of reflected object in terms of his theory of contrast. It is undoubtedly true that contrast processes play their part in the production of these phenomena, just as they play their part in every visual process, but they cannot provide a satisfactory explanation, if only for the reason that the phenomena of illumination, such as we have here, cannot be resolved into terms of contrast. Helmholtz simply overlooked the impression of changed illumination which the mirror awakens. It was probably Hering who first gave thought to the possibility of a splitting up of sensation, and he, too, later rejected it in connection with Helmholtz's experiments, and set up instead his doctrine of unity. Hering questioned not only Helmholtz's interpretation but also his facts. In his reply to Helmholtz he tried to prove that when both reflecting and reflected surfaces are perfectly uniform in colour, and when neither possesses any visible texture, the colour-impression does not split up in such a way that one surface is localized behind another. According to Hering, perfect uniformity of colour can be guaranteed only when the mirrored surfaces are small. If larger surfaces are used, the colours at the edges are different, often even complementary. In the latter case, the two colours thus seen appear as different " fragments " of the visual field, and for this reason give rise to the impression that two colours, the mirroring and the mirrored surfaces, can be seen simultaneously one behind the other in the same visual direction. It must be granted to Hering that, under the conditions he specifies, colours cannot be seen one behind the other. This, however, does not in any way invalidate the fact that such an impression can actually be had when the conditions are appropriate. Apparently even a Hering can fall into the error of sacrificing observable fact to a physical-physiological purism. It was only such an attitude as this which could make it possible for Hering to advance a doctrine of unity, which asserts that unity of colour and unity of visual direction are inseparably connected.

The fact that Fuchs [1] was successful in demonstrating how colours actually can be seen one behind another is evidence of his success in freeing himself from the attitude of the purist. Gelb's evaluation of Fuchs's experiments is worth quoting. " Fuchs accepts as his starting-point the *gestalt* psychology of Max Wertheimer. The latter had already defined the conditions under which the simultaneous presentation of two configurations one behind the other can be achieved. Fuchs proceeded to show that a convincing impression of one colour behind another can be produced when the colour which is seen and the colour through which it is seen are apprehended as two separate, phenomenally complete configurations." [2] Fuchs

---

[1] Fuchs, I.   [2] Gelb, p. 635.

showed that, when the observer adopts a critical attitude, the impression of transparency is almost always lost, because the impression of a total unified surface disappears. The more or less naïve attitude which renders the phenomenon possible is really the more natural of the two.

Bühler, too, has contributed significantly to our understanding of the problem. " The impression of two colours one behind the other," he writes,[1] " is present when certain significant cues for the duplicity are effective. These may take the form of differences in texture or other surface characteristics of the two colours, or they may come from within." " The excitations set up by each of the two processes must somehow impinge upon each other and carry each other reciprocally." One can agree with Bühler completely as long as one is not required to accept the hypothesis which he advances to explain the phenomenon, namely what he has termed the " mosaic " hypothesis. " In order to support the conclusion that the unitary retina must be capable of functioning under some circumstances as though there were two receptors inlaid in mosaic fashion, it is sufficient to presuppose two fields of organization, similar, to use a very crude analogy, to a double switch in an electrical circuit."[1] Bühler is, however, not blind to the difficulties inherent in such a mosaic hypothesis.

[1] Bühler, p. 48.

PART V

LIGHT AS SPACE-DETERMINER

§ 50. Light and Pictorial Design

The view is frequently expressed in discussions of aerial perspective that the changes in colour which directly determine localization at different distances are caused by the air. This view is incorrect; *such* changes in colour have little to do with our perception of distance. The impression of distance is mediated, rather, by the *indistinctness of objects*, the blurring of contours and the imperceptibility of fine detail induced by atmosphere. It is probable, however, that the localization of colour at a great distance and the perception of the atmosphere induced in this way have the effect of causing the actual chromatic changes, which the colours of such distant objects undergo, to recede considerably, so that they are more clearly observable through a reduction-screen than in direct vision. I shall not discuss here the changes in colour which distant objects undergo as a result of aerial perspective. They can *not* be exhausted by a reference to the reddish tinting of light objects and the bluish tinting of dark objects.

Neither the colour-value of a single object in the visual field, nor the colour-values of many objects presented together, can provide the basis for their observed orientation in space. On the contrary, the orientation of colours with reference to the observer always takes place in connection with the perception of certain spatial relationships. Orientation of objects with reference to source of light, on the other hand, is dependent directly upon certain conditions of colour and structure within the objects themselves. Equivalent clearness of surface structure leads, when objects stand at about equal distances from the light-source, to the conclusion that they are similarly orientated with reference to the light. Those parts of an object on which light is obviously superimposed must naturally be facing the light, and shadowed parts must naturally be turned away from it. Thus it may be assumed that, in general, the brighter parts of an object are turned toward and the darker parts away from the light ; it hardly ever happens that the *genuine* colours of an object are so peculiarly distributed that they compensate exactly or over-compensate for the brightness-differences resulting from the object's orientation with reference to the light. Let us suppose that we have a plaster bust, illuminated in an otherwise dark room by a light 2–3 m. away. The bust does not change its position with reference to the observer when the light is moved about the bust without any actual change in distance. The observer has, however, the impression of a changing orientation of the *light* with reference to the bust. This experience is rooted in the complex of changes induced in the colour and structure of the surface of the bust, for, even when the light-source is concealed from the observer by a screen, the impression may remain exactly the same. This experiment illustrates what we mean when we say that light is seen as passing in a particular direction through visual space or through a part of visual space. If we keep the light-source in the same position, and do the moving *ourselves*, the orientation of the bust toward the light remains unchanged, whereas it is now *our* orientation with reference to the bust which is continuously shifting. Painters sometimes use light as a method of building up the design of a picture (*Lichtführung*) ; and the same principle may be said to underlie the orientation of objects toward the light. I need not say that this effect is a fact of experience, bound up with the perception of surface colours and their illuminations, and is not in any way identical with the quality or intensity of the illumination in the visual field. The lighting effects can differ for

P

the same intensity and be the same for different intensities of illumination. The clearness with which a part of the visual field is structured in terms of light also follows the laws of field size. Sometimes the structure suggested by the light in one part of the visual field does not harmonize with that in a neighbouring part, and then we get a strange, almost uncanny impression of illumination.[1] We usually expect the light to be directed fairly clearly in a particular way, and when this is for some reason or other not the case the illumination seems strange. This was the case, for instance, when peripheral vision was cut off.[2] Everyday experience with both daylight and artificial illumination leads us as a rule to expect the direction of light to be *from above*. Lighting from below, after the fashion of footlights on the stage, may have a disturbing effect upon us. The way in which light is used as a determiner of pictorial design is a factor of extremely great importance if a picture is to be effective ; sometimes it affords the only bond of unity in a composition.

§ 51. Psychology and Pictorial Art

One of the goals of impressionism was the representation of even the most intangible, fleeting states of illuminated objects. One might very profitably begin one's study of the relationships between illumination and illuminated objects by examining the paintings of the impressionists.[3] If we wish to observe the specific colours which a painter has put upon his canvas, isolated and uninfluenced by the illumination in which the picture as a whole is standing, it is best either to approach the picture so closely that only a small area can be seen at a time or to use a kind of reduction-screen, *e.g.*, a piece of stiff paper with a small aperture in it, through which individual colours can be observed without their contexts

---

[1] *Cf.* p. 133, note. [2] *Cf.* p. 208 f.
[3] "A careful study of the paintings of the great masters . . . is of great importance for physiological optics." Helmholtz, I, p. 97.

and reduced to the prevailing illumination. The picture usually represents an illumination which is not that of the exhibition room. That this is at all possible is intelligible in the light of the fact that we can have a clear impression of an illumination of a particular quality or intensity, even when only a section of the visual field is involved. This suggests a great many questions, only a few of which I shall mention. In the first place, we find a confirmation of the first law of field size in the fact that the *more* of a picture we perceive the clearer is our impression of the illumination which the artist is representing. The colour of a small area of a picture signifies nothing in itself ; it contributes to the illumination-impression only when it is grasped as a part of the whole. This fact is important for the artist in connection with his decision as to how much of the external world is to be represented in a picture, and how large the picture is to be.[1] For the same reason, when we stand very close to the canvas the effect we get is that of the reduction of the colours of the picture to the illumination of the room, because the structure of the paint now appears in a degree of clearness which corresponds to that illumination-intensity. The colours have now lost their pictorial function ; they no longer represent objects, but appear simply as *paint* on the canvas. For every picture there is a distance from which it should be observed—a requirement which is not always respected— and failure to observe from this distance may give rise to all sorts of misinterpretation. A painting in life-size, for instance, usually demands a distance which is adequate for the object portrayed. The surface structure, too, of a represented object should appear in a proper degree of clearness. Anyone who is in the habit of paying attention to this clearness aspect will realize to what an extent the artist is forced to make use not merely of the attributes of colour-matter, but also of the attributes of surface

---

[1] *Cf.* A. Hildebrand's discussion of the dimensions used in pictorial representation (*Das Problem der Form*, 3rd ed., Strassburg, 1901, p. 78, note).

structure, if he is to attain his end. The changes induced
in the surface structure of objects by changes in illumination are of the greatest importance in the representation
of illumination conditions. In some cases the portrayal
of differences in illumination is impossible on the basis
of the attributes of colour-matter, and is to be achieved
only through the representation of structural differences.
Writers on painting often tend to assume that variations
in clearness of contour are in themselves sufficient,
without recognizing that the equally important factor of
surface structure must also be stressed. The deviations
of the structure represented in the picture from that
of its surroundings constitute the essential determinant
of the " picture atmosphere." [1] Whenever such deviations
are absent, and at the same time there are no special
colour differences to distinguish the illumination within
the picture from that without, the opposition between
picture and reality disappears. Some forms of artistic
training actually set as their goal the achievement of
such a complete illusion. True art, however, never seeks
to destroy the dividing line between what is represented
and what is real.[2] Whole periods in the history of
painting can be characterized in terms of their treatment
of surface structure. The work of such old masters as
the Van Eycks and Memling, for instance, contains a
treatment of fine detail which stands the test even of
the microscope. In such works we can always be sure
that the highest degree of surface structure will correspond to the normal illumination prevailing in the
picture. In pictures of some of the modern masters,
however, even in those which purport to represent
illumination in its normal intensity, we search in vain
for any such clear-cut surface structure ; the emphasis is
rather upon the atmosphere which surrounds the objects
depicted, and which robs them to a certain extent of their
hard-and-fast character. Clear surface structure does not

[1] Bühler includes an important discussion of the principles according to
which illumination is indicated in pictorial representation.

[2] The Wiertz Museum in Brussels contains interesting illustrative
material.

lend itself to the representation of the momentary fleeting states induced by illuminations which deviate qualitatively and quantitatively from the normal. Methods of artistic expression change in response to the demands of the material to be depicted.

§ 52. Psychology and Illuminating Technique

The technique of illumination has to do with problems of artificial control. Its immediate purpose is, thus, eminently practical. Illumination engineers have been and still are trying to free man more and more from his dependence upon the sun. They assist the eye to function effectively under conditions which would otherwise render all activity dependent on eyesight impossible. " Illumination may thus be considered as one of the most important, perhaps the most important among all the tools used by man, . . . serving as it does to increase the efficiency of all other tools." [1] The use of an artificial light-source, even when it was nothing more than the flickering, smouldering flame of a pine-torch, liberated man's life from the domination of daylight, released him, of course, too, as no other being has ever been released, from some of the beneficial restrictions which nature has placed upon his activity. Animals, for instance, are completely subject to the rhythm of night and day ; man has been able to turn night into day and day into night. The history of technical progress runs to a great extent parallel to the development of the techniques of illumination, and it would be an interesting task for the psychologist to write the story from the psychological point of view. We shall overlook this problem here, however, and turn our attention instead to the psychological questions raised by the illuminating techniques which have already been developed. Edison's invention of the electric lamp led immediately to overwhelmingly rapid developments in the field of illumination engineer-

[1] J. Teichmüller, " Lichttechnik und Psychotechnik," *Industrielle Psychotechnik*, 1925, 2, p. 198.

ing, and as a result we have everywhere almost unlimited resources for the study of the psychological problems of artificial lighting. With our present methods of producing tremendous brightnesses within very small areas, and of controlling these almost completely both as to intensity and as to spatial position, man's triumph over night has been rendered practically complete. At the same time a whole new field of investigation has separated itself out from the traditional optics, *viz.*, that of illumination engineering, a study which stands in closest relation to physiological and psychological optics. Leading illumination engineers are now willing to recognize that their science can no longer be considered as simply a branch of applied physics, as was the case in the days when it was believed that the determination of photometric values exhausted the problems of the field. It is realized now that a study of the effects of light on the human organism is equally important, so important, in fact, as to constitute a separate branch of illumination engineering. Teichmüller, for instance, has introduced the concept of " goodness " of illumination, and in doing so has recognized the importance of psychological factors. " The illumination of an open or closed space may be termed ' good,' " he writes, " when the eye is able to see surrounding objects through it clearly and without strain. This requires (1) that there be an appropriately strong illumination at every point and in almost every plane in space ; (2) that this be fairly uniformly distributed ; (3) that the lights and the various kinds of shadow be effectively distributed ; (4) that the eye be not blinded by direct reflection either from the light-source itself or from any of the illuminated objects ; and (5) that the colours of objects be clearly distinguishable and capable of being perceived, if not as easily as in daylight illumination, at least without unpleasant strain. As a last and obvious condition the lights and the illumination . . . must be stationary." It is clear from this definition that the " goodness " of an illumination is dependent on the one. hand on its practical serviceability, and on the other hand on its pleasantness, *i.e.*, on its æsthetic effect.

An illumination is good, in the practical sense of the term, when it is adapted to the activity for which it is intended. Every new performance under artificial illumination presents the illuminating engineer with a new problem. Schoolrooms, designed for reading, writing, etc., cannot be illuminated in the same way as lecture halls. In the workshop, where individuals work at special machines, different conditions have to be met, and the surgeon's operating room must be provided with a still different illumination. When we are dealing with the illumination of streets and other traffic-centres, our problem is still another one. If show-window displays are to attract the public, they must not only be clearly perceptible but must also be presented in a pleasing illumination. Thus here, as in connection with light-advertisements, certain æsthetic demands are made upon the illuminating engineer. Such purely practical problems in illuminating technique have noteworthy implications for the psychophysiology of colour. No illumination is good if it becomes so intense, as any artificial illumination may, as to produce phenomena of fatigue.[1] Fatigue effects are found most frequently when great differences in brightness produce adaptive changes in the eye, regardless of whether the eye affected be light- or dark-adapted. Any blinding effects, too, are undesirable, and should be avoided by means of frosted glass or indirect lighting. Semi-indirect and indirect light serve also to eliminate deep shadows. Contrast-relationships are useful only within limits in facilitating the perception of fine detail, although for some illumination purposes high degrees of contrast can be exceedingly useful (*e.g.*, in connection with silhouette effects). Artificial illumination always impairs the perceptibility of microstructure and of chromatic colours, and performances depending on either of these factors are best carried out in daylight illumination.

[1] *Cf.* C. E. Ferree, *Zsch. f. Sinnesphysiol.*, 1916, 49.

I have repeatedly pointed out that the psychologist has much to learn from the artist. The same source will prove fruitful for those who are interested in the use of light in architecture, to which group the illuminating engineer belongs in so far as he goes beyond his purely practical problems and concerns himself with the use of light in the creation of a pleasingly organized space. From the point of view of interior architecture, for instance, the space within a ball-room or a theatre should not merely be rendered visible, but should appear attractively organized as well. It is amazing to what an extent the whole character of a room can be influenced by the nature, the number and the distribution of the lights used and by the colour of the walls. Artists of bygone days have, in the depiction of interiors, anticipated many effects which architects have been able to produce only recently as a result of the developments in the field of artificial lighting. We find real light-architecture, however, in the construction of the old Gothic cathedrals ; for without the assistance of any artificial illumination the early workers were able so to make use of subdued daylight to achieve a genuine modelling of interior space. The modern cinema affords an excellent field for light-architecture, for here the factor of movement can be used in the modelling of space, and strikingly artistic effects are frequently achieved.[1]

[1] Further references to the psychology of lighting technique are to be found in the works of Krauss. On the physical side the best reference is O. Lummer, *Grundlagen, Ziele und Grenzen der Leuchttechnik*. Verlag Oldenbourg, 1918.

PART VI

COLOUR-CONSTANCY AND COLOUR-CONTRAST

§ 53. The Contrast Theories of Helmholtz and Hering

WE have more than once emphasized the fact that the phenomena of colour-constancy seem to be largely independent of contrast. Ever since the days of Helmholtz, however, repeated attempts have been made to bring the two fields into closer relationship with each other, and for that reason it would seem in order for us to discuss the relationship here in some detail.

The controversy between Hering and Helmholtz over the nature and origin of contrast had the effect of splitting investigators in this field into two camps, those who held to a physiological and those who held to a psychological theory. The distinction between physiological and psychological referred to the dividing line between hard-and-fast, unmodifiable, inherited factors, on the one hand, and plastic, acquired factors, capable of being influenced by individual experience, on the other. The situation might also be characterized by the statement that Hering assumed that the nervous processes corresponding to contrast were peripheral in character, whereas Helmholtz assumed them to be central. As far as the latter alternative is concerned, the attempts which recent investigators have made to determine the relative locations in the optic sector of the psychophysical processes corresponding to contrast and those corresponding to colour-constancy have met with some success.

Hering's interpretation of contrast as a special case of the interaction of retinal elements was probably one of his most fruitful contributions. Such interaction prevents the changes in photochemical or other processes, which are set up immediately by stimulation, from corresponding exactly to all changes in stimulating light. In this way simultaneous contrast enhances the sharpness of contour of objects perceived. In Hering's theory only the general facts of the interaction of retinal elements were connected with colour-constancy, not the special phenomena of simultaneous contrast. In a critique of Helmholtz's contrast theory it is best to accept v. Kries's statement of it, since, as the latter points out, " it corresponds more adequately to present-day views." [1] v. Kries holds that for some contrast-phenomena it may be necessary to assume a relative peripheral conditioning, but that others have to be accorded a central origin. In the latter case he supplements Helmholtz by assuming that for " psychical contrast " there must be a physiological correlate. Such a correlate he designates more explicitly as " intra-cortical." As examples of psychologically conditioned colour experiences, v. Kries selects the colours which accompany judgments of recognition. In this way all colour-impressions which come into being in connection with illumination must, in the final analysis, be referred to contrast. v. Kries recognizes the fact that the way in which we see the colour of a surface is in large measure independent of the intensity and wave-length of the light it reflects, and at the same time definitely dependent upon the nature and the intensity of the illumination in which it appears. The colour experiences which are brought about by illumination changes differ, however, so radically from what we are accustomed to consider contrast-phenomena that it would seem to be quite impossible to consider them as essentially the same. If I make no mistake, Helmholtz was led to consider the phenomena of contrast and the perception of illumination together because his study of illumination was confined solely to unusual cases. Thus it happened that he came to consider the perception of illumination in general as

[1] v. Kries, *Nagels Handbuch*, p. 240.

something out of the ordinary, and to rank it along with certain particularly striking cases of contrast. This view of the perception of illumination must be given up in the light of the fact that the perception of illumination is a perfectly normal process, an essential part of everyday visual perception; and on the same basis its connection with unusual cases of contrast can no longer be accepted.

Our present problem is to determine in what ways specific contrast-phenomena differ from colour experiences which may be considered as striking phenomena of colour-constancy. We have no reason to assume that people with normal colour-vision evince striking differences in connection with colour-contrast; quantitative studies of contrast seem to give distributions similar to those obtained in other quantitative studies, e.g., in the determination of colour limens. In the field of colour-constancy, however, there are enormous individual differences. Even the intra-individual differences are smaller in contrast than they are in colour-constancy. We have referred above to the lability of many of the phenomena of colour-constancy; such lability is not to be found in the field of contrast. Contrast colours weaken very little before repeated or critical observation, and are not to the same extent influenced by changes in individual set. Even such differences as these seem to me to demand that we consider the specific phenomena of contrast as essentially different from the phenomena of colour-constancy.

Such general arguments against Helmholtz's theory of contrast may be supported by means of special experiments. In the set-up described on p. 121 the disc B_2 is strongly shadowed, but the disc B_1, although it reflects the same amount of light, appears considerably darker than B_2. Let us now set up two small grey or white cardboards, C_1 and C_2, in such a way that they appear equally bright when seen against a background h, which is uniformly coloured and therefore exercises a uniform contrast influence (Fig. 12). If h is removed, B_1 and B_2

will function as contrast-inducing fields for the cardboards, C_1 and C_2. When this is performed we find that *the two cardboards remain equally bright when they are exposed to the contrasting influences of the discs, in spite of the fact that the disc B_2 appears brighter than the disc B_1.* It must be admitted that when accommodation is for C_2 the disc B_2 does not appear as bright as it does when accommodation is for B_2 itself; nevertheless the constellation is such that if there were anything at all in the nature of a psychological surface contrast, its natural effect would be to make C_2 appear darker. This experiment and variations of it with chromatic colours lead to the conclusion that, *when figural conditions are held constant, contrast effects are dependent solely on the intensity and quality of retinal excitation.*[1] A similarly negative result was obtained by Levy-Suhl in some ingenious experiments, in which he attempted to influence contrast colours by means of suggestion during hypnosis.[2] " Nowhere did our experiments reveal the influence of those psychical factors which Helmholtz assumes as the basis for his theory of simultaneous contrast; all the evidence seemed, rather, to support the assumption that there are purely physiological processes operative, which cannot be influenced by ideas and judgments in Helmholtz's sense." In the light of such observations, we are probably fairly safe in assuming that when figural conditions are held constant the phenomena of contrast are direct outcomes of the interaction of retinal elements, an interaction which is as primary a function as is their

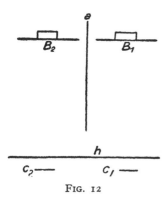

FIG. 12

---

[1] S. W. Kravkov and W. A. Paulsen-Baschmakova were able to confirm this observation. " Apparently this conclusion argues against the assumption, made by many investigators, that the mechanisms of contrast and of transformation are identical." *Psychol. Forsch.*, 1929, 12.

[2] Levy-Suhl, *Zsch. f. Psychol.*, 1909, 53.

direct reaction to light.[1] The excitations induced through contrast may affect consciousness in various ways according to the constellation of the contrasting fields. Some of Helmholtz's observations are worth repeating in this connection. He mentions, for instance, the fact that contrast effects are reduced when the contrasting fields are apprehended as independent, spatially separated objects. Similarly, in our experiments with coloured shadows and coloured illuminations, the perception of coloured illumination enhanced the phenomena of contrast. The white ground on which the coloured shadows lay appeared convincingly as chromatically illuminated. This is supported by more recent observations made by Kroh.[2]

In connection with the question as to the location of the physiological processes which underlie the phenomena of colour-constancy and of colour-contrast, I should like to report briefly G. E. Müller's most recent findings.[3] Müller formulates his conclusions somewhat as follows : 1. The contrast zone lies outside the retina. 2. The contrast zone lies before the psychophysical visual sphere. 3. The contrast zone lies before the field of binocular mixture. 4. The contrast zone lies in the visual cortex. 5. The contrast zone lies beyond the Gratiolet radiations. 6. The contrast zone lies before the zone of the " central transformation processes " (inferred from my experiments, reported on p. 236). Müller refers, too, to Th. Haack's finding [4] that " transformation affects not only the objective colours and brightnesses of circumfields but also the subjective colours and brightnesses induced by contrast in infields." Another of Müller's generalizations is also worth noting. " If central transformation is normal, but simultaneous contrast is considerably reduced or altogether absent, the deficiency is to be interpreted as follows : The contrast zone functions not as a relay station for centrally directed impulses in the optic nerve,

---

[1] Hering's view seems to be finding more and more adherents among physiologists and zoologists.
[2] O. Kroh, *Zsch. f. Sinnesphysiol.*, 1921, 52. .
[3] Müller, III, ch. 3.   [4] *Op. cit.*

but rather as the zone in which impulses coming from various points in the retina are enabled to interact by means of contrast pathways." From Jaensch's experiments on contrast in eidetic images Müller infers that the cortical excitations underlying eidetic imagery are aroused in a region which lies on the peripheral side of the contrast zone.[1]

§ 54. JAENSCH'S PARALLEL LAWS

A great many investigations, made by Jaensch and his pupils, have dealt with the relation of colour-constancy to eidetic phenomena on the one hand and to contrast on the other. Since only the latter problem will be discussed here, the literature cited below will be confined to articles dealing with colour-constancy and colour-contrast.[2] Jaensch agrees in general with my view that the phenomena of colour-constancy cannot be reduced to terms of contrast, although he holds in addition that the phenomena of contrast and those of colour-constancy "spring from a common source." In his treatment of the perception of illumination it is characteristic of Jaensch's view that coloured illumination is regarded as "abstracted." Kroh states the position somewhat more strongly. "In order that we may avoid misunderstandings," he says, "may I point out that in our use of the verb 'abstract' we are merely expressing the fact that a particular illumination is not seen." This description is quite inaccurate ; we cannot emphasize too strongly the fact that we can see all the various kinds of illumination just as positively as we see local colours. This fundamental phenomenological error has led to untenable theories. How does Jaensch come to the conclusion that colour-constancy and colour-contrast have a common origin ? He infers it from the far-reaching parallel between the laws operating in the two fields.

[1] E. R. Jaensch, *Zsch. f. Psychol.*, 1921, 87, p. 211 ff.
[2] E. R. Jaensch, *Sitzungsber. d. Ges. zur Beförderung d. g. Naturwiss. zu Marburg*, 1917 ; *Zsch. f. Psychol.*, 1920, 83 ; *Zsch. f. Sinnesphysiol.*, 1921, 52. E. R. Jaensch and E. A. Müller, *Zsch. f. Psychol.*, 1920, 83. B. Herwig, *Zsch. f. Psychol.*, 1921, 87.

" Laws of contrast become laws of transformation when in the laws of contrast the term ' circumfield ' is replaced by the term ' illuminated space.' " " The infield in contrast experiments is the field which undergoes contrast ; in transformation experiments it is the field which undergoes transformation, *i.e.*, the disc which is exposed to abnormal illumination (shadow, chromatic illumination). The contrast inducer is the circumfield, the transformation inducer the illuminated space." In keeping with this view Jaensch and E. A. Müller have formulated a law of transposition for brightness contrast and brightness transformation : " The quantitative laws of (brightness) contrast become laws of (brightness) transformation if in the contrast laws we replace the term ' circumfield ' by the term ' illuminated space.' Laws which are connected in this way have been called ' parallel laws.' The laws of chromatic contrast and chromatic transformation, like the laws of brightness contrast and brightness transformation, are parallel laws."

Jaensch's view has not won general acceptance. Some of the criticisms he aroused have been directed against particular findings, and some have been concerned with more fundamental issues. I shall permit his principal critics to speak for themselves.

G. E. Müller, referring to one pair of Jaensch's parallel laws of transformation and contrast, says : " Far from having here two parallel laws, we have rather two laws which are absolutely opposed to each other."[1] Again, in connection with the confirmation by Jaensch and E. A. Müller of my finding that colour-constancy is weaker in indirect than in direct vision, he remarks : " It is noteworthy that they have quite overlooked the question as to how simultaneous contrast in indirect vision compares with simultaneous contrast in direct vision. If they had faced this problem they would have had to recognize a still greater discrepancy between transformation and simultaneous contrast. For it is a long-established fact that contrast effects are stronger

[1] G. E. Müller, *Zsch. f. Psychol.*, 1923, 93.

in indirect than in direct vision." [1] Müller refers to the fact that a white paper appears brighter when it is placed on a black ground, and points out that in a simple phenomenon such as this, although Jaensch's principle would explain possibly why the white paper appears brighter, it could never explain how it is that at the same time the black paper appears darker. Rupp has drawn attention to the fact that contrast equations can be made fairly easily and satisfactorily, whereas in colour-constancy experiments the observer may be quite puzzled, and also to the fact that colour-constancy phenomena may disappear completely as a result of a change of attitude, particularly among painters, whereas no such effect is ever observed in the field of contrast. My own objections in this connection were based on the differences between the two fields of investigation in lability and in range of individual difference. Another very important objection raised by Müller is that when illumination is held constant a perfect equation can always be found for a contrast colour, but never for a transformed colour. He calls attention, too, to the fact that prolonged observation strengthens colour-constancy, but weakens the dark ring induced through marginal contrast about a bright field. Finally, Müller points out, the evidence indicating that the zone for colour-constancy lies behind the zone for contrast would argue against the assumption that contrast can be reduced to colour-constancy.

Bühler has dealt only briefly with Jaensch's parallel experiments. He expresses the suspicion " that the phenomena which Jaensch and E. A. Müller have been investigating are not two different things but actually the same phenomenon, that they have been comparing not the familiar phenomenon of surface contrast with illumination influences, but the same illumination phenomenon under two different sets of conditions." [2] The resulting parallels, Bühler considers, are " almost obvious."

Gelb's very penetrating criticism of Jaensch's theory follows in general the lines laid down by Bühler. Referring

---

[1] G. E. Müller, *op. cit.*, p. 7.   [2] Bühler, p. 128.

to the principle underlying the parallel experiments, Gelb says : " If the principle is applied . . . on one occasion to the study of simultaneous brightness-contrast and on another to the study of the shadowing of achromatic surface colours, it becomes immediately clear that we have no right to speak of a parallel or analogous variation of the conditions for contrast and for colour-constancy. In contrast experiments . . . it is assumed that, when any change is made in the circumfield, the infield must remain objectively constant ; it must reflect the same amount of light into the eye after the change in circumfield as it did before.   In Katz's shadow experiment, however, whenever the illumination is changed . . . the intensity of the light emitted by the shadowed disc (the infield) naturally changes at the same time ; the deeper the shadow, for example, the weaker the light coming from the disc.   In the light of such a difference in experimental conditions and experimental variations, one is forced to inquire how, in spite of the obvious parallel between the two sets of results, one has any right to infer the existence of parallel laws." [1]   Having criticized the experiments from the point of view of method, Gelb concludes as follows : " What is to be inferred from this ? Do these results . . . support the hypothesis of an essential relationship or even of a parallel relationship between contrast and colour-constancy ?   So far as we can see, Jaensch's experiments furnish no valid evidence to warrant our discussing the problem ; for a close examination of the facts makes it clear that experiments according to the method of normally illuminated equivalence discs, which Jaensch has assumed to be transformation experiments (*i.e.*, colour-constancy experiments), and to which he has opposed his contrast experiments, are not directly comparable with any colour-constancy experiments hitherto reported." [2]

Granit, too, has on the basis of his own experiments rejected Jaensch's theory.   " When, for instance, a green figure is seen at one time against a red background and

---

[1] Gelb, p. 664.   [2] *Ibid.*, p. 666.

Q

at another time in red illumination, I consider the constellations in no way—as Jaensch does—as parallel. How incorrect such an assertion would be can be seen particularly clearly in the case where the figure is barely perceptible in red illumination. The figure of the illumination constellation would in this case be iso-chromatically transformed, *i.e.*, would lose in saturation in the direction of white, while in the contrast con-stellation with maximal saturation of the background it would shine forth as a beautifully saturated green."[1]

I shall have occasion later to discuss Bühler's hypothesis that air-light has a special significance as stimulus light, and I shall show that those amounts of air-light which would have to be effective are not supraliminal. The impression of the lighting of air is co-variant with the impression of the illumination of objects; and there is no special light-stimulus to account for the impression of lighting in empty space. This fact, too, must make it evident that Jaensch's theory is not acceptable. In contrast the source of induction is clear; contrast influences come from every direction in the surroundings. In contrast, too, these surroundings themselves are changed in such a way as to produce supplementary stimuli which become effective. If, on the other hand, the objective illumination is altered, all the objects in the field then suffer a change, which is seen on the objects as a change of lighting. It is not as though a change in illumination introduced a change in air-light which became effective, while the brightness of the objects remained the same. If I am not mistaken, Jaensch could never have proposed his theory if he had not assumed— implicitly, of course—that air-light can function as an independently variable stimulus.

Since the importance of microstructure as a determinant of contrast clearness was recognized, many of the hitherto puzzling details among the phenomena of contrast have become more intelligible. Furthermore, it is now known that macrostructures

---

[1] R. Granit, *Skandinavisches Archiv f. Physiol.*, 1926, 48, p. 222.

exercise a by no means unimportant influence on contrast. Benary generalized from his experiments as follows : " The contrast effect on any one part of a configured field is not determined merely by the character, size and proximity of the other (inducing) parts of the field ; it is also of significance within which total configuration it functions as a part. Our results indicated that, for this degree of figural independence of the critical field, contrast becomes greater as a result of the inherence of the critical field in a particular whole." [1]

In many studies dealing with optical problems in painting, attention has been drawn to the significance of simultaneous contrast for the painter.   Apparently contrast assumes different rôles according to the technique selected.   Where the colour is laid in such a way that individual brush-strokes are distinguishable on the surface (*e.g.*, in the work of Franz Hals), contrast effects must be quite different from the contrast effects produced when the painted surfaces are perfectly smooth. (Most of the Dutch *genre* painters, *e.g.*, Jan Steen, Metsu and Terborch have achieved this effect.)   The painter who blends his colours together while the paints are still soft sets up quite different contrast conditions from those set up by painters who use discrete spots of colours laid side by side (*e.g.*, the *pointillistes*).   A number of important observations of the blending of chromatic and achromatic colours on the retina as a result of reduction in visual angle may be found in a study by W. v. Lempicka.[2] Prandtl,[3] in a study of hatched surfaces, reports how clear and unitary colour-impressions can be produced in the same way.

§ 55. DEPTH CONTRAST AND FLICKER CONTRAST

Bühler was the first to raise the question as to the existence of depth contrast, *i.e.*, a contrast between different depth levels.   It was probably Haack,[4] however, who first succeeded in demonstrating that the lighting

[1] W. Benary, *Psychol. Forsch.*, 1924, 5.
[2] *Zsch. f. Sinnesphysiol.*, 1919, 50.
[3] A. Prandtl, *Zsch. f. Psychol.*, 1926, 99.   [4] *Op. cit.*

of one section of space could exercise a contrast effect upon another section of space lying behind it. We may then be justified in speaking of a depth contrast as distinguished from the traditional surface contrast. Haack arranged her experiments as follows : " In front of the opening from dark-room *A* to room *B* was erected a screen, half of which was covered with velvet-black and half with white paper. In each half of this a round hole, 15 cm. in diameter, was cut. Perpendicular to this screen, and separating the black half from the white half, another screen was set up. This second screen was hung with black paper on one side and with white on the other, corresponding to the colours of the first screen, and thus producing two corners, one black and one white. The black corner was illuminated, and the enclosed space lighted, by a variable electric lamp, whereas the white corner was kept in constant shadow and received only indirect light from the walls. What was presented, then, was a very strongly lighted space bounded by black on one side and a weakly lighted space bounded by white on the other. Apart from this there were small coloured papers fastened to the black and white walls, which exercised no influence on the total brightness of the field, but which served to enhance the object character of the walls, and thereby the vividness of the impression of illumination. The intensity of the illumination was varied until the strongly illuminated black wall appeared through a reduction-screen as equal to the weakly illuminated white wall, *i.e.*, until both walls reflected exactly the same amount of light." The observers looked through the two openings, and at the same time, of course, through the differently lighted sections of space in front of them, into the room *B*. No fixation-point was used, the observer's eye being permitted to rove about at will. This is an important fact, because, whereas surface contrast is strongest when the eyes are held stationary, depth contrast is clearest when observation is roving. What, then, was the nature of the impression produced ? Through the opening in the weakly illuminated white wall everything in room B appeared normally clear and normally bright. Through the opening in the strongly illuminated black wall, however, room B appeared very much darker, as though it were filled with dark smoke or mist. Several other differences were observable, but I shall not discuss them here. Haack tried analogous experiments with chromatic illumination and chromatic colours, but was unable to produce any clear-cut differences in the illumination of B or in any other aspects of the impression it produced. Haack has as yet made no attempt at a thoroughgoing explanation of depth contrast. "We have no other alternative," she writes, "than to distinguish this [depth contrast] for the time being from the physiologically determined bi-dimensional contrast, and emphasize the impossibility of its explanation in physiological terms, and to recognize positively the existence of a psychological contrast between differently illuminated or lighted spaces."

Flicker contrast refers to the contrast effects induced by flicker in surfaces which are objectively quite free from flicker. Haack made a study of the extent to which flicker contrast obeys the two laws of field size. She reports that "in connection with the experiments performed under the conditions of the first law of field size, although the contrast effects proved to be definitely dependent upon the size of the infield, they did not, nevertheless, follow that law exactly. . . . Now the fact that the first and second laws of field size were not found to hold for such labile and easily influenced conditions as those of flicker contrast may be accepted as further support for the assumption that they hold only for . . . phenomena of colour-constancy and not for phenomena of contrast." [1]

Haack made a further study of the effects of variation of illumination intensity on (1) simple brightness contrast; (2) marginal contrast; (3) chromatic brightness contrast; and (4) chromatic contrast. Her results indicated that contrast-phenomena are almost completely

[1] *Op. cit.*, p. 124.

independent of the intensity of illumination, even when the latter is varied within wide limits, thus distinguishing themselves markedly from phenomena of colour-constancy, whose very existence depends upon illumination. "We have here contributed a few more important facts toward the clarification of the relationship between contrast and transformation, and their implication is that contrast is to be regarded as fundamentally different from transformation." "The colours and brightnesses induced by contrast function altogether as object colours, inasmuch as they tend to remain constant even when the illumination is very greatly reduced (to approximately 1/180 of itself)." [1]

Haack has demonstrated that a real or apparent increase in the size of the surface undergoing contrast involves no change which follows the laws of field size. Thus we have here, too, an essential deviation from the behaviour of colour-constancy phenomena, for it was in terms of the latter phenomena that the laws of field size were formulated. There is, then, no ground for Jaensch's assumption that colour-constancy and colour-contrast follow parallel laws.

§ 56. The Modes of Appearance of Negative After-Images

May I add here a few remarks about successive contrast, in so far as this expresses itself in negative after-images. Let us suppose that we have two equally large chromatic or achromatic papers appearing in different chromatic or achromatic illuminations, but so chosen that when reduced they appear exactly the same. If, now, we fixate the two papers (unreduced) for the same length of time, and project the resultant negative after-images on the same background, we shall find that these differ neither in mode of appearance nor in hue, brightness and saturation. The same holds true for colours which differ in mode of appearance but appear equal after reduction.

[1] *Op. cit.*, p. 127.

Haack performed experiments of this nature, using surface colours, film colours, volume colours, lustrous colours and luminous colours. By means of an episcotister she made sure that each of the original colours possessed approximately the same light-intensity. The after-images were projected on a paper surface in a dark-room. Under these conditions, she found it impossible to distinguish clearly between the after-images of colours differing in mode of appearance. The same result was obtained, moreover, by Braddock in a repetition of some of my own observations.[1] Haack explains her results by referring to the absence of clearly perceptible structure in after-images. The structure of the original colour is not reproduced in the after-image, since the colour differences carrying the microstructure are far too small. In confirming this, Haack ran a number of fruitful control experiments. "The objects used were equal squares of wood, cardboard, leather and woollen cloth, and care was taken in their selection that they were as nearly equal as possible in hue and brightness. A comparison of the four corresponding after-images revealed no differences in appearance. All four looked the same, and were similarly uniform and undifferentiated. The details of structure and the differences in the colouring of the micromorphic parts are too small to be reproduced in the after-image. Eye-movements do not cause the microstructure, on the basis of which the material of objects is recognized, to disappear ; after-images, on the other hand, follow every movement of the eyes, and in doing so undergo change." With the sacrifice of microstructure, the after-image loses the capacity for expressing the differences between surface colour, film colour and volume colour. Lustre can appear only in connection with surface colours, and if a colour is to be luminous it has to shine forth so much more strongly than the colours about it that it can never be represented in an after-image.

[1] C. C. Braddock, *Amer. J. Psychol.*, 1924, 30.

PART VII

MEASURES OF THE PERCEPTION OF ILLUMINATION

§ 57. General Remarks

All the experiments so far reported have dealt with the equation of surface colours which differed in quality and intensity of illumination. The illuminations and the differences between them were perceived as such, but they were not themselves treated as objects for comparison. Now all these experiments can be reversed in such a way that *the illuminations are accepted as comparison objects, and the colours of the objects which they enclose are " abstracted."* Quantitative studies can then be made of equivalent illuminations, of liminal and supraliminal differences, and of any other attributes of the illuminations to be compared.

§ 58. Quantitative Studies

The first experiments on differential sensitivity to illumination were made by Krüger.[1] " In the first experiment two black episcotisters . . . were set side by side at a distance of about 25 cm. from each other. Practically no light was reflected directly by either. The observer looked successively through the episcotisters at the same room behind them and at the same landscape visible through an open window. The opening of one episcotister was kept constant (standard value) and the other was varied (comparison value) according to the method of limits . . . in the attempt to determine the threshold values for the impressions of illumination

[1] H. Krüger, *Zsch. f. Psychol.*, 96, 1924.

248

created by the episcotisters. . . . The observers were explicitly instructed to take the illumination of the whole visual field into account. In parallel experiments with Maxwell discs (both under the same illumination) . . . the differential sensitivity for greys was determined according to the method of limits." The opening in the standard episcotister was kept at 180°, and the corresponding Maxwell disc was set at 180° white and 180° black. I shall include the first of Krüger's tables. The first column contains the liminal values for the Maxwell discs M, the second those for the episcotisters E, and the third the quotients Q obtained by dividing E by M.

Observer	M	E	Q
Ka . . .	5·9	15·9	2·7
Ke . . .	4·9	22·5	5·0
Ra . . .	6·4	21·2	3·3
Er . . .	4·1	8·9	2·2
Bo . . .	2·2	9·8	4·5

Two interesting facts emerge from these results. The first is of fundamental importance, namely that a really quantitative study of differential sensitivity can be carried out just as well with illumination impressions as with the brightnesses of surfaces in the same illumination. In the second place, the difference limen proves to be very much higher for illumination than for surface brightness, for the quotients are all greater than one, ranging from 2·2 to 5·0. Here we have quantitative support for the observation, reported in § 14, that changes in illumination intensity may easily escape notice, at least more easily than changes in brightness of surface colour.

In another series of experiments, Krüger compared the limen for *change* of illumination impression with the limen for change of surface brightness. Here, too, the limen proved to be higher for illumination than for brightness. Krüger connects this result with the fact that in everyday life surface colours hardly ever undergo local changes which are independent of changes in illumination.

Kardos,[1] in his experiments on the perception of illumination, limited himself to a relatively small section of the visual field, and since his observations took place in artificial illumination, the conditions did not in general favour clearness in the phenomena. His study makes it still clearer, however, that quantitative experimentation with perceived illuminations is possible.

[1] L. Kardos, *Zsch. f. Psychol.*, 1928, 108.

PART VIII

COLOUR-CONSTANCY AND THE PROBLEM
OF DEVELOPMENT

§ 59. ANIMALS

WITHIN the field of developmental psychology it is customary to include animal psychology, the psychology of childhood and adolescence, folk psychology, some branches of psychopathology, and some branches of the psychology of abnormal conscious states (*e.g.*, dreams). The psychological study of animals, children and adolescents has contributed significantly to our understanding of colour-constancy. We have already reported the relevant material from pathology, and the information at our disposal related to the modes of appearance of colour in dreams.

The first experiments on colour-constancy in animals were performed by Köhler with chimpanzees and hens.[1] Köhler trained hens to pick grains from the brighter of two papers, both of which lay in moderate illumination. In the crucial experiment, the darker paper was placed in direct sunlight, where it undoubtedly reflected more light than the other; nevertheless, the hens chose the paper which reflected less light, *i.e.*, the paper which was " really " brighter. The same result was obtained in experiments with chimpanzees, in which case the animals had to distinguish on the basis of brightness between boxes filled with fruit. Köhler rejects the suggestion that the colour-constancy evinced by these animals might have been due to individual experience, and asserts that in explaining this kind of vision we must make one of

[1] W. Köhler, *Abh. d. preuss. Akad. d. Wiss., Math.-phys. Kl.*, 1915, 3 ; *Zsch. f. Psychol.*, 1917, 77.

two alternative assumptions. We have to do here either with an inherited function, " which, because of its biological significance, has been acquired and fixed, and which is now transmitted as something essentially complete ; or, on the other hand, with a type of vision, which is biologically very appropriate, of course, but in the acquisition of which experience and natural advantage have played no essential part—a type of vision resulting from a development of the visual apparatus in response to external and internal conditions, which, quite apart from the biological advantages involved, made such a development inevitable."

Köhler used only illuminations with which his animals were undoubtedly familiar, and never any explicit chromatic illuminations. For this reason, one is naturally not prepared to assert that in Köhler's experiments " individual experience " played no rôle. There is still less ground for such an assertion, however, in connection with certain experiments with hens performed by Katz and Révész.[1] Here the illuminations were chromatic, and undoubtedly quite foreign to the animals. The behaviour of the animals under these conditions can be rendered intelligible only by the assumption that even in chromatic illumination there is a certain constancy of colour. When highly coloured and white grains of rice are scattered before hens, the white grains will almost always be selected first. On the basis of this discrimination, it is very easy to train hens not to touch any of the coloured grains. " After the hens had been trained to reject all coloured grains a parallel experiment was arranged. White grains of rice were scattered on a white floor, and the white floor was then illuminated so strongly with chromatic light, e.g., blue or yellow, that through a reduction-screen it appeared at least as highly saturated as the blue or yellow of the coloured grains. . . . Hens were now placed before the illuminated grains, and in spite of the fact that they had rejected pigmented grains of the same hue and saturation, they ate the

[1] *Zsch. f. angew. Psychol.*, 1921, 18.

illuminated grains without any hesitation. It must accordingly be assumed that the chromatically illuminated grains created an impression different from that created by the pigmented grains." [1]

It is probable that the retina of the chimpanzee differs little from that of man, and the hen's retina is known to be particularly well supplied with cones. It would accordingly be interesting to extend the experiments on colour-constancy to animals whose vision is predominantly rod vision, such as fish. Such experiments were performed by Burkamp with various kinds of cyprinidae. [2] We know now, as a result of v. Frisch's experiments, that fish are by no means colour-blind, as v. Hess had believed. Without such a postulate, there would be no point in experimenting on fish with chromatic colours and chromatic illuminations. Burkamp observed behaviour in his fish which led to the conclusion that fish show colour-constancy phenomena, not only when illumination is varied in intensity, but also when chromatic and uncommon illuminations are used.

Even the strict behaviourist would have to admit, in the light of these experiments, that visual situations in which the animal behaves in the same way are more closely related to each other than are those in which he behaves in different ways. To put it more concretely, a weakly illuminated white must bear a closer relationship to a normally illuminated white than to a strongly illuminated black. We have no right here to speak of genuine partial equations, after the analogy of the partial equations in the corresponding experiments with humans. Such partial equations are probably possible only in situations in which colours are apprehended categorically, *e.g.*, where words or other symbols for the colours are available.

At one time I held that the phenomena of colour-constancy are to be expected only in connection with cone-vision, because only by means of cones is it possible

[1] *Op. cit.*, p. 320.
[2] W. Burkamp, *Zsch. f. Sinnesphysiol.*, 1923, 55.

for us to perceive microstructure. I still hold that precise surface colours are perceived only when microstructure is perceptible, and that illumination is never more clearly given than when it is connected with a clearly visible microstructure. We may conclude, however, from Gelb's report of his patient (whose vision might possibly be considered as resembling most closely that of the normal individual with dark-adapted eyes), and from other sources, that the phenomena of colour-constancy may within certain limits be independent both of micro-structure and of cone-vision. When we bear in mind the fact that Burkamp's experiments were performed under conditions of rod-vision, his results become par-ticularly significant. I have already drawn attention to the fact that we may have phenomena of colour-constancy in peripheral vision if the eye is light-adapted, and if the stimulated areas are large enough we may have them even when the total retina is dark-adapted. Thus we may conclude that there is a certain constancy of colour even in human rod-vision.

Bühler remarks in one place that " after the analogy of the illumination-factor, which is involved in our present differentiated perceptions, we must conceive of the most primitive visual impressions of lower animals in such a way as to recognize in day and night, bright and dark, the first dimension of developing vision." [1]

§ 60. CHILDREN

If colour-constancy develops during the course of the life of the individual, we should be able to learn something about it from experiments with children. I made the first experiments of this kind with children from three to eight years of age, and came to the conclusion that " the numerical results of the experiments showed no significant deviations from those derived from experiments with adults." In the study cited above, Brunswik set for himself the task of studying the development in childhood

[1] K. Bühler, *Psychol. Forsch.*, 1925, 5, p. 182.

of the perception of albedo. Beginning with children of three years, he included in his experiments samples of all ages up to adulthood. The technique he used was that of illumination perspective. Brunswik, too, succeeded in demonstrating the existence of a fairly high degree of colour-constancy, even in his youngest subjects. He believed that he had also found evidence of a development in colour-constancy with increasing age, the curve reaching its peak as a rule between the ages of eight and fifteen, and then sinking. In my review of his work I have pointed out that Brunswik's results can lay no claim to general validity, since they are very closely bound up with the experimental technique he employed. Burzlaff succeeded in showing that, if a suitable technique is employed, children can display a colour-constancy which is almost ideal, and which is in no way inferior to that of adults. The most suitable technique is method D described above (§ 30). I shall give only the average brightness-quotients which he found for his youngest children, aged four.

Colour value :

360°	321°	270°	210°	183°	135°	90°	40°	20°

Quotient :

1·00	0·98	0·98	0·93	0·95	0·98	1·03	1·02	0·97

We can see that all the brightness-quotients lie in the neighbourhood of one, some higher, some lower. Here we are obviously justified in accepting the highest values as our point of departure, since they show that in children almost ideal colour-constancy can exist. In those cases in which the result is not obtained, the deviations are to be attributed to the experimental conditions. Thus it would appear that within the age-limits so far studied there is no evidence of any particular development of colour-constancy.

Is it likely that, during the ages which Brunswik and Burzlaff did not study, the perception of albedo undergoes a development ? Or are we to assume that as soon as the visual apparatus functions after birth, it functions essentially as it does in adult life, responding to incoming stimuli with the whole range of modes of appearance and with the phenomena of colour-constancy ?   No one, I believe, can assert positively that the colour-vision of the child undergoes no development at all.   In our discussion of individual differences we have indicated how certain attitudes toward colour, to which we have become habituated, may lead to a change in colour-perception. It might be contended that in the same way the colour impressions which we receive undergo certain general changes with increasing age, corresponding to the develop-ment of certain attitudes ;   or stated perhaps more correctly, that our attitudes toward objects undergo changes, and these in turn involve changes in the colour-impressions which we receive.   May I refer back to my discussion of the distinction between subjective and objective attitudes,[1] in which I pointed out that the shift from one attitude to another may affect not merely the phenomena of colour-constancy but also the mode of appearance itself of a colour.   If it could be assumed that during the first years of life the child's perceptual attitude undergoes a transition from the subjective to the objective, we might be justified in speaking of a development of colour-constancy in the child.   Not long ago, such an assumption might easily have been made.   Present-day psychology, however, with its biological emphasis, would be inclined to challenge it.   The subjective attitude is theoretical and unnatural, whereas the objective attitude refers directly to objects.   As soon as the child has any kind of commerce at all with subjects, he loses himself completely in his activity, and shows no tendency to degrade them to the status of mere visual phenomena. As a matter of fact, no matter how hard we try, we can never succeed in inducing the child to shift from a practical to a theoretical attitude, and to consider objects simply as bits of colour.   This would argue against the hypothesis of a development of colour-constancy in the

[1] *Cf.* § 33.

individual. On the other hand, I should not dare to assert *a priori* that the child sees in exactly the same way as an adult sees. In the pre-linguistic period this could not be true, because during this period colours are not apprehended as belonging to specific categories, and the significance of categorical apprehension for colour-constancy has already been emphasized. A further assumption might be that the child has from the beginning the same kind of object-experience as the adult. This is improbable, at least during the period before the child has learned to manipulate objects with his hands. How do things appear to the child during the period before his hands have become active ? Child psychology has as yet given us no answer to the question. Anyone who refuses to content himself with cheap hypotheses must recognize that as yet child psychology has failed to make any significant contribution to the problem of the development of colour-constancy or of the modes of appearance of colour.

One might expect that the reports of cases in which the blind have been made to see by means of operations would throw some light upon this problem. I have searched the literature, however, and found no relevant information.

§ 61. EIDETICS

According to Feyerabend,[1] an eidetic image of a chromatically illuminated surface can be produced and projected like any other eidetic image on a screen. He concludes from his observations that " there is an agreement between the colours of the infield of the eidetic image and the colour displayed by the infield in ordinary vision when transformation processes are operative." [2] Feyerabend holds that by virtue of its projection upon a neutral ground, the eidetic image succeeds in liberating the processes involved in transformation from a connection in which they are always found in ordinary

[1] *Zsch. f. Psychol.*, 1924, 94 ; 1924, 95.
[2] *Op. cit.*, p. 233.

experiments.[1] There are, he suggests, two possible ways of interpreting the relationship between transformation and eidetic imagery. (a) " The transformation of the colour of abnormally illuminated objects depends upon the operation of the same counter-process as that which operates in the objectively neutral infield in a negative eidetic image." (b) " The transformation of the colour of abnormally illuminated objects can be traced genetically to the operation of a counter-process, which appeared earlier in the eidetic stage of development, and which gives rise in adolescent eidetics . . . to complementary eidetic images." [2] Following Jaensch, Feyerabend adopts the second, or genetic, view. " We must," he thinks, " interpret [the phenomena] which Hering has termed the interaction of retinal elements and adaptation, and in terms of which he explains contrast and colour-constancy, . . . as processes belonging to early stages in colour-vision, which during the course of development have become fixed as sensory reflexes, and which are still observable in tangible form in the eidetic phenomena of adolescence, . . . expressing themselves in the form of negative eidetic images. These negative eidetic images thus represent a genetically early stage of what later appears as the complementary colouring observable in objectively neutral infields during transformation." [3] In further experiments, Feyerabend produced complementary eidetic images both of illumination colours and of retinally equivalent surface colours, and found that in complementary eidetic imagery the phenomena behave in essentially the same way as they do in ordinary vision.

Some other observations, made by Feyerabend, are worth noting. Eidetic images of illuminations were projected, sometimes on homogeneous surfaces and sometimes on objects. " Anything which strengthened the apprehension of a seen colour as object contributed to the desaturation of the eidetic image at that point," i.e., functioned as a condition of higher colour-constancy.

---

[1] *Op. cit.*, p. 234.   [2] *Op. cit.*, p. 246.
[3] *Op. cit.*, p. 247.

When eidetic subjects are shown, in normal illumination, the objects upon which the eidetic images of chromatic illuminations are later to be projected, a higher degree of colour-constancy results. If three objects appear in the eidetic image as coloured and one of these (a white object, for instance) is removed, presented in normal illumination and then returned to its place with the other two, the latter two will continue to appear coloured, while the first will appear white. There are still other ways in which recent experience may influence the eidetic image of an illumination, but these need not be mentioned here. Such observations are closely related to the fleeting memory-colours which we have already described.

PART IX

THEORIES OF COLOUR-CONSTANCY

§ 62. HELMHOLTZ, VON KRIES AND HERING

In recent years there has been a growing interest in the history of the problem of colour-constancy, and for this reason I shall devote some pages here to historical discussion. Fortunately, I am able to draw upon the article by Gelb, with whose position I am in large measure in agreement.

"Helmholtz developed his empiristic theory of perception under the influence of certain philosophical ideas centring about the concept of 'construction,' which were rooted in the thinking of the middle nineteenth century. The principal thesis of the empiristic doctrine is as follows: Our sensations are 'signs for external things and processes, which we must learn through experience and practice to interpret.' Being signs rather than 'representations,' our sensations can, of course, in no way resemble the physical processes which elicit them. They correspond, however, to the physical stimuli in strict, point to point fashion, and such sensations are for Helmholtz genetically as well as actually prior; they precede perception. Perceptions are not, however, like sensations, original, but represent 'higher' processes. They are ways in which we have learned to understand our sensations."[1] Now how, according to Helmholtz, do we succeed in interpreting our sensations when the illumination is changed? We do so by measuring the light reflected from objects according to a different standard. "Seeing as we do the same coloured objects under . . . different illuminations, we learn how to

[1] Gelb, p. 603.

construct, in spite of the differences in illumination, a correct idea of the colours of the objects, *i.e.*, we learn to judge how such an object would appear in white illumination, and since it is only the permanent colour of the object which interests us we become quite unconscious of the individual sensations upon which our judgment is based."[1] " A grey paper in sunshine [may] be brighter than a white paper in shadow ; nevertheless we see the first as grey and the second as white, because we know very well that if the white sheet were placed in sunshine it would appear much brighter than the grey does at present."[2] Hering's reply to this view of Helmholtz's is well known. " Since . . . it is only on the basis of the colours of the things that we see that we could come to that knowledge of the illumination which is to serve as our standard of judgment, and since, on the other hand, it is exactly these colours which are supposed to be the resultant of such a judgment, the theory we have just described moves in a fruitless circle."[3] Gelb has risen to the defence of Helmholtz against Hering's accusation. " Since Hering did not recognize Helmholtz's distinction between sensation and perception, his suggestion that Helmholtz had been arguing in a circle is not altogether convincing. v. Kries has already pointed this out. He notes the fact that Hering speaks unhesitatingly of the colours ' in which we see objects,' whereby the word ' see ' might refer to either ' sensation ' or ' perception ' in Helmholtz's sense. Helmholtz finds the bases for our estimates of illumination only in what we ' sense,' whereas our estimates of illumination function as determinants of what through a process of judgment we ' perceive.' "[4] Gelb summarizes Helmholtz's theory as follows : " According to this point of view, the phenomena of colour-constancy represent the product of an ' unconscious influence of judgment.' When, for instance, a weakly illuminated white paper and a strongly illuminated black reflect physically equal amounts of

[1] Helmholtz, II, p. 243 f.   [2] *Ibid.*, p. 110.
[3] Hering, VI, p. 20.   [4] Gelb, p. 608.

light, the sensations, Helmholtz would say, are also the same. As a result of practice and experience they are, however, differently interpreted, *i.e.*, we have in the two cases different ideas or perceptions."[1]   Helmholtz's theory is difficult to reconcile not only with the rich phenomenology of human colour-perception but also with the results which animal experiments have yielded. [2]

Helmholtz's theory of contrast constitutes an indispensable component of his general theory of perception, and v. Kries has revised and developed the latter just as he has the former. We may describe his contribution in Gelb's words :   " J. v. Kries concedes, it is true, that a strongly illuminated black paper may produce the impression of black, and that an adjacent shadowed white, reflecting objectively the same amount of light, may produce the impression of white. Nevertheless, he holds that the sensations are in the two cases the same. Sensation and object colour are, in fact, two quite different things, and under some circumstances they may not agree with each other, since our impression of the constitution of a seen object has come into being ' in a different and more complicated way' than have the corresponding sensations. v. Kries does not consider it possible to explain the higher perceptual processes in terms of ' unconscious' judgments and inferences. Perception, too, is to be regarded ' as the immediate, irresistible outcome of physiological processes' ; but it represents the outcome of a composite process, of a physiological mechanism which is composed of two parts or phases in such a way that the mode of combination of these parts is not fixed, but is comparable rather to the alternative connections of a multiple switch." " We can see how Helmholtz's distinction between sensation and perception reappears in v. Kries in the form of a physiological hypothesis, the ' switch' theory; how here, too, isolated, strictly stimulus-determined and unmodified sensations are held to constitute the original foundation or raw

[1] Gelb, p. 603.   [2] *Cf.* § 59.

material for genetically later and higher forms of organismic reaction."[1] v. Kries's interpretation of Hering's classical shadow experiment affords us a good illustration of his view. " When the impression shifts from that of spot to that of shadow, there can be no doubt that something in it or on it remains unchanged throughout. We may characterize this most appropriately by saying that the sensation as such has remained unchanged, while its association with empirical concepts has undergone a peculiar modification. But what term are we to use for this constant element, if we use the word ' sensation ' for its association with the concepts of white and grey, *i.e.*, for spot and shadow, and speak of the reversal as a change in sensation ? "[2] Now it seems to me that the significant thing about the reversal is not that this or that empirical concept is associated with a " constant sensation." What is essential is not the external association which is formed. On the contrary, the very fact that, when we attempt to characterize the impression in words, one term is appropriate at one time and another at another, according to the circumstances, would presuppose original differences in the impression. This and similar differences can undoubtedly be perceived by children long before they are capable of forming concepts, a fact which could be proved by behaviouristic methods. Indeed, it is highly probable that the same could be demonstrated for animals.

Let us turn now to Hering's attempts to explain colourconstancy. According to him, practically all the work is done by physical (pupillary) and physiological adaptive mechanisms (interaction of retinal elements). As a result of their operation, he holds, a chromatically or achromatically coloured object affects the eye in the same or approximately the same way when the illumination changes in quality or intensity. " Hering, however, exaggerates the influence of retinal adaptation and of

---

[1] Gelb, p. 604.
[2] Supplement by v. Kries in Helmholtz, *Physiologische Optik*, 3rd ed., 1910, vol. 3, p. 491.

variations in pupillary size, and his assertion that the subjective brightnesses of objects remain approximately constant contradicts the most common of everyday experiences."[1] We have pointed out on more than one occasion that the results of our experiments cannot be explained in terms either of pupillary function or of retinal adaptation. Paradoxical as it may at first sound, such a thoroughgoing efficiency on the part of the adaptive mechanisms as Hering postulates is not even to be considered as desirable ; for it would partially or wholly compensate for any change in illumination, and thereby make it imperceptible. It is simply a fact which we cannot deny that we see achromatic and chromatic changes in illumination, provided they overstep certain limits, and that at any time we are able to give a fairly good report of the prevailing illumination. If Hering were right, how could we ever see those indubitable modifications of surface colours which can come into being only as consequences of changes in quality and intensity of illumination ? In comparison with the peripheral adaptive mechanisms, " psychological " factors play, according to Hering, a relatively unimportant rôle in preserving the constancy of colour of seen things. Such factors operate through the medium of *memory colours*. Memory colour, as Hering defines it, is not to be lightly identified with the *genuine* colour of an object. Hering assumes, rather, that the object has already been seen several times, and that in this way its individual memory colour has been built up. Where the objects with which we are dealing do not possess specific natural colours as do blood, coal and snow, we can build up memory colours for them only as they become familiar to us as this or that particular hat, table, glove, etc. Usually the individual objects belonging to a particular class possess no such uniform, artificial colouring as to render it possible for us to infer with any degree of certainty from the individual object to its genuine

---

[1] G. E. Müller, *Zur Grundlegung der Psychophysik.*   Berlin, 1878, p. 419.

colour. In the light of these considerations, I cannot see how " memory colours " can play any rôle in our perception of objects which are individually unfamiliar to us and which are presented under varied conditions of illumination. It frequently happens that the objects themselves are less easily recognizable than are their colours. Certainly there was no memory colour attached to the papers which we used in our experiments, for there is nothing in the essence of paper to suggest black, white or any other colour, and the papers which we used were distinguished by no marks which could serve to arouse any particular memory colours in the observers. Thus I cannot assign any great importance to memory colour in connection either with our experiments or with colour-constancy in general. In my opinion, the adaptive factors to which Hering refers are effective primarily in the struggle with the insufficiency of the dioptric apparatus in the production of sharp contours, and thus they contribute indirectly to the reliable recognition of surface colours in a changing illumination, rather than bring about the constancy of colour according to the direct method mentioned by Hering. The significance of the interaction of retinal elements for the elimination of the false light and the sharpening of contours has been so adequately discussed by Hering [1] that there is nothing to be added. That pupillary adjustment may be considered as serving the same function has also been suggested.[2] One might even assert with some justification that in certain cases the interaction of retinal elements is actually a *hindrance* to the recognition of colours. Against a bright sky a white flag-pole or a white window-frame will appear grey or black. Cases such as these, in which surface contrast disturbs the recognition of objects, confront us in whichever direction we turn.[3]

[1] Hering, VI, p. 151 ff.
[2] *Cf.* F. Schenck, *Nagels Handbuch*, p. 79 f.
[3] C. v. Hess has shown how, if the circumfield is brightened, contrast may under some circumstances render differences in light-intensity of 1 : 800 imperceptible. *Pflügers Arch.*, 1920, 179.

§ 63. Bühler

The first section (*Space and Colour*) of Bühler's work begins with a critical examination of Berkeley's argument against the assumption of a primary, stimulus-determined perception of depth. Bühler introduces into his discussion v. Kries's view that the portions of space lying between objects lack sensory character, but that the idea of space (in Kant's sense) is a unitary and invariable element of our consciousness. "Visual space as a total unity actually exists and appears in perception, not, however, merely as a scheme devoid of sensory content, but as a medium filled with brightness; and furthermore, this brightness is stimulus-determined. If we are successful in proving that scattered air-light is physiologically effective, and that visual space (which is often called "empty") is filled with the resulting brightness, we shall be better able to do justice to the facts brought forward by v. Kries and many others than we should be by simply applying Kant's doctrine of the *a priori* character of perceived space in the form which we have criticized." According to Bühler, the air-light, *i.e.*, the light which is reflected by the particles of dust and gas in the air, not only represents in a general sense the stimulus for the perception of empty space, creating empty space, as it were, but also determines the impression of illumination in any part of space. Bühler bases this theory, which is fundamental for his entire work, almost exclusively upon L. Weber's investigations of the albedo of air-particles.[1]

I have tested experimentally the significance of air-light for the impression of illumination. The results indicate that with clear atmospheric conditions the light from a stratum of air which is not too thick lies below the limen for the light-adapted eye, and for any intensity of illumination having practical significance. Under these conditions, air-light is physiologically irrelevant. The light of a fog may fill space, but then the fog we see is

---

[1] L. Weber, "Die Albedo des Luftplanktons," *Annalen der Physik*, 1916, 4. Folge, 51.

seen in an empty space which is itself filled with brightness. Before I describe my own investigations of air-light, I shall pursue Bühler's ideas a little further. We ask with Bühler : " How is it possible to find in homogeneous air anything for the eyes to fasten upon to make the parallax effective, even if only slight distances are involved ? " Bühler leaves this question unanswered, although it is impossible to maintain the air-light theory without a completely satisfactory solution of the problem. From our point of view, the perception of brightness in the space of a glass bell exhausted of air does not, as it does for Bühler, constitute a problem. Bühler mentions that according to Hering the perception of so-called empty space between oneself and the objects one sees is quite different in daylight from what it is at night. Bühler now assumes that Hering believed he could see the brightness of the air directly. This assumption is, however, hardly admissible, for Hering was undoubtedly thinking of brightness and darkness in this context in the phenomenological and not in the physical sense.

Bühler describes the following hypothetical experiment to test as satisfactorily as possible the ability of the eye to take account of conditions of illumination. " Let us imagine two similar spherical chambers as large as rooms, one of which is painted black and the other white. Now let us imagine that the observer's eye is at the centre of each sphere, and that the illumination (*e.g.*, from a point-source light above his head) is so regulated that just as much (white) light per unit area is reflected to the eye from the walls of the one sphere as from those of the other. Furthermore, the two surfaces should be without any visible (shadow-casting or shadowed) texture and without any shading in the visual field. The question is whether this eye would be able to distinguish (*e.g.*, by successive comparison) the one wall as a more weakly illuminated white from the other as a more strongly illuminated black or dark grey. A photographic apparatus cannot do this, but perhaps the human eye might succeed under certain conditions. The problem is to determine under what conditions and by means of what resources this might be possible." I should like to remark, in connection with this hypothetical experiment, that Bühler has so defined all the conditions affecting the perception of albedo and illumination that it is impossible to see which of these could be varied. If we take the conditions as Bühler has defined them, then we may say that the eye will *not* be able to distinguish between the two walls. Bühler supposes that " our knowledge would be significantly richer if this experiment were carried from the realm of imagination to that of reality." The predictable result, however, must shatter such a hope.

Now how, according to Bühler, is the perception of albedo formed independently of change of illumination ? " Let us assume that the light-waves reaching the eye are not the only radiations at the time, but that the air in front of and around the object is likewise radiating light, and in such a way that the eye notes this. The intensity of this air-light should be directly dependent upon and an expression of the intensity of illumination prevailing in the space and lighting the object. Then the air-light so operative might provide the measure we are seeking, and the achromatic colour of the object might stand out, according to its albedo, from the perceived brightness of the air. According to such an hypothesis, what could not be learned directly from the arrangement of objects could be learned indirectly from another source. We should then have a simple and technically elegant substitute for the whole balancing of object colour and illumination, a substitute for the determinative quotient—intensity of reflection/intensity of illumination." I have demonstrated experimentally that, owing to its low intensity, the air-light cannot have the function which Bühler claims for it. The experiment was performed in a room with a wall standing in approximately normal illumination. Near the wall an easily movable tunnel-like arrangement, about 50 cm. long, was placed in such a way that it did not cast a shadow upon the wall. Therefore the wall reflected just as much light to the observer's eye when the tunnel was in place as when it was removed. A white paper introduced into the tunnel seemed, after reduction, to be decidedly darker than a normally illuminated black paper. This indicates that the air-particles in the tunnel were almost completely deprived of light. In front of the tunnel we set up a screen with a fairly large opening. An observer sitting in front of it could see the wall of the room and the space in front of it, but could not see the walls of the tunnel at all. Now, as regards the impression of the wall and its illumination and of the illumination of the empty space in front of it, it made no discoverable difference whether the tunnel was in place or moved aside. In both cases, the observer saw the wall and the empty space in front of it in approximately normal illumination. If the intensity of air-light really determined the perceived brightness of the empty space and the illumination of the objects lying behind it, the empty space should appear to be filled with darkness, and the impression of the illumination of the wall should be entirely different in the observations through the tunnel, since almost the entire layer of air-particles lying between observer and object is then deprived of its light. Since neither is the case, even this simple experiment seems to show that air-light has no perceptible influence either upon the brightness of empty space or upon the illumination of objects. We shall now report an experiment which is to a certain extent a reversal of the one just described, and which points to the same conclusion. The observer looked through an opening in a cardboard at a large movable paper screen, which, together with the empty space lying in front of it, appeared to be normally illuminated. Then, without changing noticeably the distance of the screen from the observer, we turned the screen a little away from the light, so that it and the space in front of it were perceived in diminished illumination. The layer of air between the observer and the screen was not deprived of its light by this procedure. Yet this light was not in the least able to maintain the apparent brightness of the empty space at its previous level or to influence measurably the apparent illumination of the wall. Repetition of these experiments with chromatic illuminations likewise showed the insignificance of the air-light in these cases.

The results of these experiments justify us in concluding that the light of *thin* layers of clear air lies below the sensory limen for the human eye, and hence cannot in any way play the rôle given to it in Bühler's theory. It seemed wise, however, to fortify our results by a quantitative procedure, even though this gave only approximate values. The experiment was performed in the courtyard of the laboratory on a clear, bright day, when the sky was lightly clouded. We selected from a series of grey papers two whose respective equivalents on the colour-wheel were 21° white and 23° white. From the brighter paper we cut two pieces respectively 3 and 60 mm. square, and pasted them concentrically upon two pieces of the darker paper, respectively 10 and 200 mm. square. When the smaller of these stimulus-objects was seen from a distance of 30 cm. (*i.e.*, through a layer of air of the same thickness) the brighter paper was just distinguishable from its background. Since the difference was continuously noticeable, the " limen " obtained in this way was a little higher than it would have been if it had been obtained by the method of limits, yet only a moderate increase of light upon figure and ground (the same increase of light upon both) was sufficient to make them indistinguishable. The slight cloudiness produced in a glass vessel of water by adding a small quantity of milk was sufficient to obliterate completely the difference in brightness between figure and ground. Now we come to the second step of the experiment. The larger stimulus-object was seen from a distance of 6 m. At this distance the factors of retinal projection and contrast were the same as in the case of the smaller stimulus-object. The layer of air between the observer and the object was, however, about twenty times as thick as before. What was the effect ? The figure stood out just as well as in the case of the smaller stimulus-object.

Yet even when I stood at a distance as great as 45 m. from the object (the greatest distance which I was able to use) the figure was just as distinguishable as before. Therefore the light of a layer of air 45 m. thick has not the slightest influence upon a limen, as we have determined it, and is not as potent as a thin layer of weakly clouded liquid. How can the light of a layer of air 30 cm. thick have a measurable influence upon visual perception, in the two ways mentioned by Bühler, when it can exercise no influence upon a limen even when this thickness is multiplied by 150 ? The experiment shows that air-light may be neglected as a stimulus up to distances of at least 45 m. Obviously if the distance were multiplied by a few thousand, even the tiny amounts of light reflected by the air-particles in this experiment might become effective. We may note here expressly that with a distance of several kilometres the air-light does become effective, and may give rise to phenomena of aerial perspective.

We may insert here a brief discussion of an apparently remote phenomenon—the so-called Aubert-Förster phenomenon. This name is given to the observation that objects of greater apparent size are not apprehended as well as objects of less apparent size, even though the retinal images are equally large. Many investigators have sought physical explanations of the phenomenon. It is hardly an accident, however, that no investigator of the phenomenon has succeeded in explaining satisfactorily how air-light could make the more remote object less perceptible. The fact that the Aubert-Förster phenomenon can be demonstrated only by most exact methods may be considered another argument against the air-light theory.

We can increase artificially the light-content of the air by increasing the number of light-bearing particles in the air. We may produce a thick smoke in a dark-room by means of a cigarette, for example, and illuminate it by the cone of light from a projection apparatus. If we look from near-by, we see bright lines of smoke streaming through dark space ; from some distance away we see a unitary bright strip with the mode of appearance of film colour tending toward volume colour. We have no impression of an empty space filled with brightness, although the theory we are attacking here would lead us to expect this result. Even if a fog, which supplies considerable air-light, gathers in the open air, the empty space does not appear brighter. We see instead whitish fog in space which has itself lost its glassy, clear brightness, and the objects behind the fog appear veiled and less strongly illuminated.

We shall call attention to a final fact which can be reconciled to the air-light theory only with great difficulty. In § 22 we mentioned the changes in the impression of illumination accompanying micropsy in the Koster phenomenon. Since there is no objective change in air-light in micropsy experiments, it is difficult to see how the air-light theory can explain the change of illumination actually observed.

Now if air-light does not provide the stimulus-basis for the impression of illumination of empty space, how can such an impression arise in such a compelling way ? We may answer, as we have already indicated in § 7, that in the lighting of empty space we have a *phenomenon of co-variance*. The lighting of empty space corresponds to the illumination of the objects enclosing and bounding it. We have already discussed in several other connections how space is coloured when the mode of illumination of these objects is not unitary. Empty space possesses unlimited capacity for adapting itself to the colour of the prevailing illumination. It offers no resistance, and readily submits to any type of lighting. Why is this so ? Because it has so little strength as a bearer of colour. We might say that its optical inertia is so low that it follows readily any directive optical force, however slight it may be, that comes into the situation. That would not be so if empty space had at its disposal independent optical energies of its own, *i.e.*, if the light of air-particles had any relevance. We arrive, therefore, at

an hypothesis which is directly opposed to Bühler's :
We can understand the facts concerning the lighting of
empty space only by assuming that air-light is a negligible
quantity, if it does not extend through too great a
distance.

Bühler's duplicity theory, which has been emphasized
more by Bühler's students than by Bühler himself,
appears in three different forms : (1) the air-light
theory; (2) a form supported by v. Kries's classical
duplicity theory (the perception of local colours being
attributed to the cones, and the perception of air-
light to the rods) ; and (3) the theory based upon the
scattered light in the eye (the so-called " false " light).
I believe that what I have already pointed out is sufficient
to show that the first two of these forms of the duplicity
theory are untenable. As for the third form, I have
remarked in a review that I can find no connection between
scattered light in the eye and this new hypothesis concerning the significance of air-light. In his answer to
my review, Bühler said that this seemed unintelligible
to him. " There is scattered light both outside and
inside the eye. Yet I hesitate even now to complete the
analogy by saying *expressis verbis* that the two are similar
in effect." Bühler thus finds it self-evident that the
scattered light in the eye originates in scattered air-light.
This statement, however, not only lacks self-evidence,
but is incorrect. Scattered " false " light is found in the
eye under all conditions, whether or not light of air-
particles reaches the eye, since its cause is turbidity of
media in the eye, especially of the vitreous humour.
Yet whatever its source may be, it is impossible to
segregate it immediately in perception and treat it as
a separate factor. The only reason why I have explicitly
discussed these matters again in this connection is that
Brunswik and Kardos[1] have criticized me for not
considering the true value of this form of the duplicity
theory.

S. Krauss is one of Bühler's students who have accepted

[1] *Zsch. f. Psychol.*, 1929, III.

the air-light theory as a starting-point.[1] According to Krauss, it seems, the rods perceive the brightness of the air, and thus provide the measure for colour-constancy. After what we have said, it is unnecessary to discuss this point of view again. Bocksch[2] also accepts Bühler's air-light theory.

Of all the students of Bühler, Kardos has adhered most tenaciously to the air-light theory.[3] It is difficult to understand how an investigator who advocates the duplicity theory with particular emphasis can question the phenomenal character of illumination. " I· contend that ordinarily we do not see illumination in the strict sense, even though we make judgments about it with astounding immediacy. Careful introspection shows that when we are in a well-lighted room we see nothing except objects. Their degrees of clearness and pronouncedness provide the basis for our prompt judgment about the illumination, but the latter is not necessarily a separate palpable content of consciousness." Kardos[4] writes as follows about my experiments on air-light : " Although the experiments performed by Katz to test this assumption [i.e., that air-light lies above the physiological limen] might well give rise to some reflection, the possibility that air-light lies above the physiological limen is far from being excluded." He adds to this general formulation the statement that " the perception of shadow and of luminous objects "[5] provides a satisfactory confirmation of the air-light hypothesis ; but he brings forward no proof of this statement. It has been found, on the contrary, that there may be impressions of shadowing and of luminosity when the influence of air-light is entirely excluded. Shadows may be perceived when the less strongly illuminated layer of air is only a few millimetres thick and cannot possibly have physiological

[1] Zsch. f. Psychol., 1926, 100 ; Pflügers Arch., 1926, 212 ; Zsch. f. Sinnesphysiol., 1926, 57 ; Ber. ü. d. X. Kong. f. exper. Psychol., Jena, 1928 ; Arch. f. d. ges. Psychol., 1928, 62. Also H. Bocksch and S. Krauss, Zsch. f. Psychol., 1926, 99.
[2] H. Bocksch, Zsch. f. Psychol., 1927, 102.
[3] L. Kardos, Zsch. f. Psychol., 1928, 108.
[4] L. Kardos, Bühler Festschrift., Jena, 1929.   [5] Op. cit., p. 62.

importance ; and there are luminous surfaces, *e.g.*, a faintly luminous plate of milk-glass, in front of which we cannot see even a trace of air-light.

Together with Brunswik, Kardos[1] has again expressed himself on the duplicity principle. Here we find references to " Bühler's pure duplicity principle," which purports to lead beyond the three forms discussed above. What is the strict formulation of this pure duplicity principle ? It rests upon the assumption that " sensory experience is determined by something in addition to the waves reflected by the surfaces, and the difference between the two psychical effects is connected with a difference in this second factor." " It is evident that the difference in that factor (*which we cannot yet identify specifically*) must be parallel to the difference in the illumination at the time, so that this second factor is a single-valued function of the illumination." This formulation of the pure duplicity principle is so general that it permits us to place under it all the theories hitherto proposed. In their search for the unknown factor, Brunswik and Kardos come close to my own view of the significance of the total insistence of the visual field for the formation of the phenomena which we have been considering. The relationship is, in fact, so close that the factor which they are seeking, instead of being an unknown, is one which has been known for some time.

§ 64. GELB

Gelb begins his consideration of the principles underlying colour-constancy by declaring himself in agreement with my criticism of Hering. He agrees both with my view that the perception of surface colour and the perception of specific illumination are essentially related, and with my finding that all colours undergo an undeniable change whenever a change in their illumination becomes visible. From this point Gelb proceeds as follows : " Meanwhile this very finding, as well as the problematical

[1] E. Brunswik and L. Kardos, *Zsch. f. Psychol.*, 1929, 111.

association of visibility of illumination with perception of surface colour . . . remained in Katz's theory without exercising any recognizable influence upon it. Dominated probably by the traditional problem of the discrepancy between stimulus and colour reaction, he too was led to an empiristic explanation of his results. While he holds that the colour-impressions which objects in normal illumination give us are for the time being capable of no further explanation, and thus assigns a unique position both descriptively and genetically to normally illuminated or genuine colours, he considers the impressions yielded by objects in non-normal illumina-tions . . . as acquired through experience. He assumes that here, in non-normal illumination, a central trans-formation becomes effective, which makes the colours appear as though they were in their normally illuminated or genuine state."[1] I am in thorough agreement with Gelb's anti-empiristic arguments. I no longer use the concept of transformation in its earlier sense, and I share Gelb's view that " the perception of surface colours in normal illumination is no less and no more a problem than is their perception in non-normal illumination."[2] As I have already explained, I no longer assign a special genetic position to normal illumination, although I still insist that normal illumination is, as I have described, phenomenologically distinct from all others. It is bound up with the clearest perception of microstructures, and, among other things, it furnishes an important basis for the experience of specific quantities and qualities of illumination, a fact which Gelb does not consider in detail in his discussion.

Gelb's central position may be stated in his own words. " ' Severance of illumination and that which is illu-minated ' and ' perception of a resistant and definitely coloured surface ' are two different expressions of one and the same fundamental process. This process takes place in such a way that colour-impressions which are co-ordinated with one perfectly specific phenomenal

---

[1] Gelb, p. 671.   [2] *Ibid.*, p. 672.

illumination can never belong in exactly the same way to another phenomenally given illumination. Thus, for example, to every perceived illumination intensity there is co-ordinated a specific white surface. Accordingly a white surface undergoes a change in pronouncedness and liveliness (Katz) with every change in illumination intensity. Furthermore, Katz's experiments have also shown that a blue surface in reddish-yellow illumination, for instance, will never appear exactly the same . . . as a blue surface in another illumination. Is it possible, in the light of these facts, to ask the traditional question as to how visual objects retain their colour appearances in spite of changes in quality and intensity of illumination ? Apparently not." " The problem of colour-constancy ceases herewith to be that of explaining a discrepancy between stimulus and seen colour, and becomes a part of the general problem of the structure of the visual world. The phenomenal severance of illumination and illuminated object . . . is simply an expression of a particular way in which the visual world is structured. . . . Our visual world is not built up through the operation of accessory, higher (central, psychological) processes upon an original raw material . . . composed of stimulus-determined and unmodified primary sensations. The sensorium is constituted, rather, in such a way that at any time we are confronted with a world of things which, according to the existing external stimulus constellation and internal set, may be articulated and configured in any one of a great many different ways. This articulation and configuration is essentially related to such factors as visibility of a specific illumination, perceptibility of clear-cut surfaces and complexity of organization in the visual field. Such factors are, as we have seen, indispensable conditions of the appearance of colour-constancy phenomena." [1] I am in complete agreement with this general discussion, too, partly because of the very fact that it is so general. In some places I cannot agree with Gelb's specific applications of his point of view, but, to avoid

[1] Gelb, p. 672 f.

destroying the unity of his presentation, I have dealt with these minor differences of interpretation in connection with the specific experimental results with which they are associated. The most important place in which I have disagreed with Gelb is in § 31, where the significance of the articulation of the visual field for colour-constancy is discussed. There I drew attention to the fact that the articulation of the visual field cannot in itself provide a basis for the apprehension of the quality and intensity of the illumination in the visual field. This part of Gelb's theory requires supplementation, and this I shall attempt to provide in my discussion of the total insistence of the visual field. Finally, the theory must be supplemented also with reference to the question as to how we can effect a synthesis of the innumerable specific illuminations which we see and the colours which we see in these illuminations.

§ 65. The Total Insistence of the Visual Field

What determines the impression of illumination ? What enables us to speak of a normal, high or low illumination in the visual field ? In order that an impression of normal illumination be had, it is sufficient that the objects in the visual field be clearly perceptible in every detail of their structure. The fact, however, that clearness of surface structure may suffer either from an increase or from a decrease in illumination intensity, without involving any loss in our ability to pass judgments upon the illumination, renders it evident that clearness of surface structure is not the sole determinant of the impression of illumination, and forces us to look for a criterion of illumination intensity which is relatively independent of the clearness factor. Our observations of surface colours seen behind volume colours indicate plainly that the same degrees of blurredness may accompany impressions both of heightened and of diminished illumination. Were we to succeed in demonstrating the existence of a factor which, in relative independence of clearness of

surface structure, determined the impression of illumination, we should have to assume that this factor was *always
effective*, *i.e.*, even when the illumination appeared normal.

I should like now to suggest that under ordinary
conditions a visual field whose illumination is approximately uniform possesses for all intensities of illumination
a total insistence; that it is this total insistence which
determines the particular illumination intensity which
we perceive; and that upon this total insistence the
quality and pronouncedness of the colours in the visual
field depend. If, other conditions being equal, a high
total insistence is present, we have the impression of
strong illumination; if it is low, the illumination we see
is weak.[1] Granted that such a factor as that of total
insistence exists, it becomes a no more puzzling problem
to understand how the impression of illumination intensity can be derived from degrees of insistence than it
is to understand how a colour of a particular albedo in
a particular illumination can be judged as white, grey,
etc. So far as the absolute judgment of an illumination
prevailing in the visual field is concerned, we have to
postulate an absolute memory for that particular degree
of insistence. The experiments on the insistence of
variously illuminated surface colours [2] indicated that the
eye feels itself equally affected when it receives approximately equal amounts of light. Thus it is not particularly
difficult to compare the insistences of colours which
belong to differently illuminated visual fields. We may
assume that the degrees of insistence which permit of
comparison are effective not merely under the controlled
conditions of comparison but also in our everyday
observation of colours when we are not instructing
ourselves to compare. Now it is time to consider in
greater detail what we mean by total insistence.

---

[1] Absolute memory for colours is very great. This has been demonstrated in Westphal's study of the immediate judgment of primary colours
(*Zsch. f. Sinnesphysiol.*, 1909, 44) and in a similar study by Lotte v. Kries
and Elizabeth Schottelius of colours other than the primary colours (*Zsch.
f. Psychol.*, 1909, 42).

[2] *Cf.* § 21.

v. Kries remarked in one place : " It seems correct to assume that the impression of an object as white, grey, etc., is determined not merely by the brightness of the sensation aroused by its retinal image, but also to a great extent by the impression which we receive of the illumination in which the object is standing. The latter, however, is in general determined by the brightness in which at the same time we see other objects around it. Thus an object appears as white, bright grey, etc., not, or at any rate not solely, on the basis of the sensation it arouses, but also on the basis of the relationship which this brightness bears to that of the whole visual field, and more specifically to that of its immediate surroundings." [1]   It is possible that here v. Kries had in mind a factor analogous to our total insistence.

By the insistence of a colour we usually understand the strength with which it bores its way into consciousness. I contend that the visual field as a whole also has the capacity to besiege consciousness with different degrees of forcefulness. It is easy to determine total insistence when the whole visual field is artificially illuminated in a uniform way, but more difficult when the illumination is irregular. If the diffuse and complicated articulation of the normal visual field renders it difficult for one to obtain a clear experience of total insistence, one can make the observation easier by looking through a glass which disturbs accommodation in such a way as to make everything appear in dispersion circles. Such a glass prevents sharp contours or specific areas from standing out clearly. The greater the uniformity with which we apprehend the individual parts of the visual field, the more readily we achieve the impression of total insistence. If we look through an episcotister at any ordinary visual field, we can produce a great many different degrees of total insistence by varying the size of the episcotister opening. A limiting case is reached when the episcotister is entirely closed. The visual field has then an objective intensity of illumination of zero, and the colour-impression has reached its lowest degree of insistence, *i.e.*,

[1] v. Kries, *Nagels Handbuch*, p. 239.

subjective grey. As the episcotister is opened, total insistence increases. At the same time certain parts of the visual field become brighter and more insistent, and certain other parts *may* become darker and less insistent. Occasionally small parts of the visual field may quite accidentally retain the insistence of the subjective grey. The total insistence of any visual field, no matter how it is illuminated, increases continuously as the episcotister opening is enlarged. The upper limit of this is simply the strongest perceptible intensity of illumination. If throughout life we were to be presented with a visual field which was filled out in one particular way, we should have no difficulty in believing that total insistence determined the impression of illumination at any particular time. But we must face the fact that in reality the visual field is filled with all sorts of different objects, coloured in all sorts of different ways. Must we not assume that, corresponding to the innumerable ways in which the visual field can be filled, there must be equally numerous degrees of total insistence ? And must not this number be so great as to destroy any secure basis for the rooting of illumination impression in total insistence ? I believe that if we succeed in proving that in ordinary life total insistence is far more dependent upon *changes in illumination* than upon any possible changes in the *colours of the objects filling the visual field*, we may answer the question in the negative ; for the question which faces us is how we can obtain an impression of the prevailing illumination intensity, no matter what that intensity may be, and no matter what objects happen to be filling the visual field. The following discussion will serve to answer this question. The maximal brightness-differences which occur in the colours of everyday life are smaller than we might tend to think. In our experiments the brightness-ratio of the velvet-black to the white was about 1 : 60. Also we seldom encounter natural object colours as deep as this black, and the range of brightnesses within which the objects in our surroundings fall is very much smaller than that ordinarily used in the laboratory.[1] According to our experiments on the range of sensitivity of the normally adapted eye (§ 38), we can reduce the illumination of a white paper to about 1/360 of normal illumination without causing its brightness to change essentially. Thus, even in such illuminations, we are probably able to perceive surface colours and to recognize them with some degree of certainty. On the other hand, I found that the illumination in midday sunlight was at least a hundred times as intense as that used in our experiments. We may consequently assume that the intensity of the illumination in which we are accustomed to observe and to judge the objects about us varies within the approximate limits of 1 : 36,000.[2] This range is to be compared with the range of 1 : 60, within which variation in the amount of light affecting the eye may, *even in extreme cases*, be accounted for on the basis of variations in object colour alone, *with illumination held constant*. Let us assume for the moment that the whole visual field is filled with objects of the brightness of our white paper, and is normally illuminated. If, now, the illumination were made more than sixty times as intense, the total insistence would be heightened *even if* at the moment at which the illumination was strengthened all the white colours were replaced by velvet-black. On the other hand, if a normally illuminated visual field were filled with black objects, and its illumination were then reduced more than sixtyfold, the impression of weakened illumination would persist even if all the blacks were replaced by whites. In reality, however, the consciousness of illumination never has to overcome such " unfavourable " constellations of object colour. The colours of the objects about us seldom belong to the extremes of the brightness

---

[1] The remission factor of new-fallen snow is probably no greater than that of our white paper ; and, on the other hand, I cannot remember ever having encountered objects in nature which reflected less light than our velvet-black.

[2] " It has been found that the light of the sun is 800,000 times as strong as the brightest light of the full moon " (Helmholtz, I, p. 108). Thus the lower limit which we have assumed for our range of illuminations is about twenty times as strong as full moonlight.

scale, and even when they do they hardly ever constitute the dominant colours in the visual field. Since the colours of the objects in our customary surroundings—in our room, on the street, in the open landscape—vary within relatively narrow limits, we may consider the brightness-changes induced in the visual field by changes in the genuine colour of its objects as *relatively constant in degree* as compared with the brightness-changes induced by modifications of illumination intensity. We shall consider total insistence as the determining factor in our judgments of the prevailing illumination only in so far as it seems to offer an adequate explanation for the degrees of illumination actually distinguished. Krüger's experiments have shown that our sensitivity to differences in illumination is great enough to render such an accomplishment possible. To summarize our conclusions from the foregoing discussion, we may say : *Total insistence is so very much more dependent upon the intensity of the illumination than it is upon the colour of the objects which fill the visual field that it may be quite readily accepted as the basis for the absolute judgment of the illumination intensity at any particular time.*

That total insistence may be the factor determining the impression of illumination intensity is quite comprehensible. But how does it function in the assignment of quality and pronouncedness to the various subordinate wholes in the visual field ? How does it happen, for instance, that the same partial insistence of a visual area may under the influence of one total insistence give rise to the sensation of grey and under the influence of another total insistence give rise to the sensation of white ? In answering this question, we must naturally forsake the purely phenomenological method and have recourse to measurement. We have already taken a few steps in this direction (particularly in Part III) in those experiments in which we determined what relationship two light-intensities must bear to each other if in different illuminations they are to arouse the same impression of quality (in different degrees of pronouncedness). Experimental procedures such as those developed by Metzger in his study of the total field might very readily lead to the determination of numerical values for total insistence to supplement our present more qualitative approach.

Total insistence does not function merely as a determinant of the quality and pronouncedness of the surface colours of a visual field, but it also determines within broad limits which intensities of light are to produce impression of *luminosity, glow and lustre.* This is immediately evident in the light of the fact that in every visual field, however it may be illuminated, the arousal of these impressions depends upon the amount of light reflected by the brightest surfaces of the field.

In advancing the hypothesis about the rôle of total insistence formulated on p. 279, we made the reservation that all the different parts of the visual field must be illuminated in approximately uniform fashion. We may now consider this reservation in somewhat greater detail. The perception and judgment of the intensity with which a certain section of the outer world, *e.g.*, a house with some surrounding objects and an area of sky above it, is illuminated is practically independent of the amount of sky perceived above the house. We can verify this by standing at an appropriate distance from the house and raising our eyes from the bottom to the roof, in this way increasing the amount of sky present in the visual field. It can be shown that the apprehension of the illumination of the house and its surroundings, based on the insistence of their colours, does not owe its existence merely to the fact that the sky appears as film colour, in which there is no distinction between illumination and that which is illuminated, and not as a surface colour. The illumination would be apprehended even if the sky, without changing in insistence, were to appear as a surface colour. For, according to the laws of field size, *different* impressions of illumination can be had at the same time in *different* parts of the visual field, and this takes place under conditions which are fulfilled in the case of the

normally illuminated house. If a difference in degree
of insistence between two parts of the visual field is to
be apprehended as a difference in illumination, it must
exceed a certain minimum. Within areas which seem
equally strongly illuminated, those factors which indicate
object character (surface structure, contours, etc.)
appear in approximately the same degree of clearness.
When areas appear as differently illuminated, the differences in clearness have exceeded a certain limit. It might
seem as though this difference, being more noticeable,
were more important for the *distinguishing* of differently
illuminated areas, than are differences in insistence.
Impressions of illumination which differ only with respect
to clearness of structure, and not with respect to insistence, can be produced experimentally. Between our
eyes and the objects at which we are looking we can
bring a glass vessel, filled with a turbid fluid which has
been so selected that what is seen through it possesses
approximately the same insistence as that possessed by
the other parts of the visual field. Since the surface
structure of the objects seen through the vessel is blurred,
the objects appear as though immersed in fog. The
degrees of insistence present within the various parts of
the visual field must be held responsible for our apprehension of the way in which those parts are illuminated.
In so far as the insistence of a particular part of the
visual field determines the illumination seen in it, it also
determines the quality and pronouncedness of the surface
colours which it contains. The different degrees of
clearness with which the impression of a particular
illumination within a particular area is had follows the
two laws of field size.

A small section of the external world can deviate very
easily from equally illuminated surroundings with respect
to the insistence of its surface colours or the clearness of
it surface structure. When such is the case, judgments
of its colour are determined according to its albedo and
the intensity of the prevailing illumination. The difference in clearness of surface structure simply has the

effect of causing its structural relationships to be apprehended in a different way. It might happen, however,
that all the parts of a large sector of the external world
deviated in the same direction from the rest of the
visual field with respect to quality and insistence of
surface colour and to clearness of surface structure. If
such were the case, these deviations would not be apprehended simply as changes in genuine colour and in
structure within an unchanged illumination. They would
be seen, rather, as outcomes of a change in the intensity
of the illumination within that sector. Thus, within the
totality of the visual field there are subordinate totalities
which follow their own laws. The clearness with which
a sub-totality appears as such varies directly as the size
of that sector of the external world which is subjected to
such changes in insistence of colour and clearness of
surface structure. When distance localization is held
constant, the size of the perceived sector of the external
world varies directly as the size of the retinal area affected.
When retinal size is held constant, it varies directly as
the distance at which it is localized. Thus the two laws
of field size are intelligible in terms of the same principle.

§ 66. When can we see Chromatic Illuminations ?

In the foregoing section we explained how it is that
we can succeed in judging correctly the *intensity* of an
illumination, even when the objects undergo great
changes in brightness, and consequently reflect considerably more or considerably less light. Our judgments
of illumination intensity are, in other words, almost
completely independent of the brightness of the colours
filling the visual field. We are now faced with an analogous
question : How are correct judgments of chromatic
illumination possible, when the visual field is usually
filled with *chromatic* surface colours, which in *normal*
illumination reflect the same kind and intensity of light
as that reflected by *achromatic* surface colours in *chromatic*
illumination ? This question may not, of course, be

answered simply by a reference to the fact[1] that normal illumination prevails most of the time, and for this reason takes precedence over chromatic illumination. That would explain only why normal illumination is determinative for the *genuine* colours of an object, leaving unanswered the question as to how the immediate perception of a certain illumination as red, green, etc., is possible. The following considerations may throw some light upon the question. When the visual field is flooded with daylight, it never happens under normal conditions that all visible objects are definitely tinged with a single chromatic colour as they are when the whole visual field is subjected to the same chromatic illumination; nor does it ever happen in daylight illumination that those parts of the visual field which possess a highly saturated chromatic colour display this colour *in every tiny detail* of their surfaces, as they do in chromatic illumination. As I recall all the ways in which, outside the laboratory and in normal illumination, the visual field is usually filled with objects, I can think of none in which all objects are uniformly tinged with the same colour. Even if one were to try to create such a situation experimentally, one would encounter great difficulties. One would, for instance, have to use a fairly large surface, located at some distance from the eye, and either completely or almost completely filling out the visual field. The " tiny details " mentioned above would also have to be taken into account. A chromatic *film colour* presents a uniformity of colouring which is never found in a surface colour. Even the coloured papers which we use in experiments, and which are more uniform than most of the surfaces we see in everyday life, possess a microstructure which in daylight shows certain chromatic irregularities. Such irregularities are most pronounced in white daylight illumination. In chromatic illumination they are less clear, and if the chromatic illumination is very intense, the micro-elements may fuse together almost completely. In the obliteration of microstructure

[1] *Cf.* p. 90.

through chromatic illumination, it makes no difference what hue is possessed by the paper or by the illumination. Now as soon as such an impression is produced, *viz.*, that of a uniform tinting of the visual field and of a fusion of the irregularities of colour, the colour seen ceases to refer altogether to quality and saturation of surface colour, and is experienced in part as chromatic illumination. The impression of chromatic illumination is clearest when the whole visual field undergoes such changes. The clearness of the impression depends upon the size of the visual area involved in exactly the same way as does the clearness with which changes in illumination *intensity* are seen. Chromatic changes of this kind can be induced in surface colours (when fairly large parts of the visual field are involved) only through changes in the quality of the *illumination*. In our previous discussion we showed how total insistence functions in the determination both of the intensity of the illumination seen in the visual field and of the way in which the visual field is articulated. The present discussion has shown how the articulation of the visual field may depend as well upon the quality and intensity of a perceived chromatic illumination. Cases in which surface colour is perceived in *complementary* illumination do not, it seems to me, require an explanation which differs from that for cases in which the relationship is not complementary.

It is possible for us to have the impression of a *new* illumination quality, one which has never before been experienced, without having first observed the various changes which this illumination brings about in various colours. This fact is of considerable significance for an understanding of the nervous mechanism which constitutes the basis of the impression of any particular illumination quality or of the resulting judgments of colours in the visual field. Our observations of colours in intense chromatic illumination[1] have some bearing upon this problem. Let us assume that someone has hitherto seen surface colours only in *qualitatively normal*

---

[1] *Cf.* p. 193 f.

illumination, and is now presented for the first time in his life with a visual field which is chromatically illuminated, and which is filled with surface colours arranged in an unfamiliar way. It is quite probable that, even under these conditions, he will apprehend *this chromatic illumination as such*, and will perceive the surface colours in keeping with this illumination.

In the experiments reported on p. 187 ff., almost the whole visual field (in which disc *A* lay), and in the rest of the experiments reported, only a relatively small part of the visual field was chromatically illuminated. Because of the chromatic illumination, the surface colours perceived did not appear in their full saturation. They appeared, in fact, as considerably less saturated than when they underwent reduction to a qualitatively normal illumination. The effectiveness of a chromatic illumination is not confined to those situations in which the illumination as such is clearly recognized. It may exercise an influence upon our judgments of colour even when it is not recognized as such. A somewhat faint chromatic illumination which fills the whole visual field may, in fact, be recognizable as such only after considerable practice.

§ 67. The Synthesis of Illuminations

The theoretical discussion of § 65 closed with the suggestion that we consider how we effect the synthesis of the innumerable specific illuminations which we see and the colours which we see in these illuminations. We have immediate knowledge of the fact that all possible experiences of illumination are essentially related to each other, and are interchangeable with each other. There are no islands of illumination impression to which no bridges from other such impressions lead. How can it be that we have this unity within multiplicity, and what are its consequences ? For the sake of simplicity, I shall confine myself in what follows to changes in achromatic illumination, *i.e.*, to variations in illumination intensity.

T

The conclusions can be carried over without any difficulty into the field of chromatic illuminations.

Within limits there belong to every specifically illuminated visual field a specific white, a specific grey, a specific black, etc. Perhaps we shall have to accept this simply as a fact which is capable of no further explanation. Is this equivalent to an admission at the same time that we have no ultimate explanation, either, for the fact that the same qualities in differently illuminated fields are co-ordinated with each other, white with white, grey with grey, black with black, etc.—co-ordinated, that is, in the sense that, when the illumination of the visual field is changed, the white (grey, black, etc.) of the first illumination becomes " the same " white (grey, black, etc.) of the second ? All our experiments were concerned with the setting of such equations. In practical life, too, however, we are daily and hourly effecting such visual co-ordinations, even if they are not carried out with the solemnity and accuracy of the laboratory. When we open a drawer and select from its weakly illuminated interior a white paper which matches the white paper on the table, we have effected such a co-ordination. The housewife accomplishes the same thing when in a poorly lighted shop she picks out some material which matches in hue and brightness some material which she keeps in her well-lighted bedroom. Is it to be assumed that in all such co-ordinations the translation of an impression belonging to one illumination into the corresponding impression belonging to another has already been consciously performed on some previous occasion; or at least that such translations have been experienced in connection with individual colour-impressions, and these individual experiences built up into schemata which function for new impressions ? The question is not easy to answer. It need hardly be said that even an affirmative answer would not signify a return to an empiristic interpretation of colour-constancy ; for we are concerned here not with the resolution of one colour-impression into terms of some standard impression, but rather with the emergence of a superordinate unity as a result of the linking together of several colour-impressions of the same order. It is definitely a psychological, not a psycho-physical, issue, for the problem would arise even if there were no colour-constancy. In spite of the fact that a negative answer seems to be indicated by the experiments with animals, particularly those of Katz and Révész, I am still unready to accept such an interpretation. Even if our visual centres, and those of the animals which have been studied, were so constructed that the organism required no previous experience to be capable of such co-ordinative performances, such experience is, never-theless, constantly being had, and it must lead inevitably to regular co-ordinations. It would be somewhat strange, in fact, if this experience were of no consequence for our vision. Fluctuations of daylight, changes in artificial illumination, the movement of an object from one room to another—all are occasions on which we experience the transition from one illumination to another, and all provide situations in which different illuminations are seen together and colours are seen to undergo corre-sponding changes in pronouncedness. A final answer to the question formulated above is not prerequisite to a discussion of the significance which actual experiences of transition have for the synthesis of illuminations, and for our belief in the invariance of the colours of objects. Here empiristic speculation is still of some value, even if it is to some extent this very approach which forces us to relinquish the old concept of association and adopt instead the new concept of chain-association. It is only the latter concept which can do justice to such a peculiar intertwining relationship as that which obtains between illumination and illuminated object.

The most compelling reason for the recognition of illumination as one of the factors rendering possible the perception of objects must lie in the experienced fact that in total darkness objects disappear completely from visual perception, although we continue to be aware of their existence, primarily through the medium of touch.

An object is called into being by illumination, without ceasing to exist when the illumination is removed. At one time I inclined toward the view that tactual-kinæsthetic experience played a part in the constitution even of the detailed aspects of the phenomena with which we are here concerned. Now I am not so sure that this can be proved. In § 2 I called attention to the experience of " visual resistance " aroused by surface colour. I do not think that this is simply carried over from the field of touch. To me it seems much more probable that such phenomena as those of colour-constancy would be found even in a being which possessed visual organization similar to ours, but lacked touch. Without disparaging in the least the intimate relationship which exists between the visual and the tactual, I should be unwilling to assume that it is only touch which makes such phenomena possible. It is quite likely, however, that this relationship may be of significance for the development of object consciousness, and may in this way contribute indirectly to colour-constancy.[1]

Sometimes the objects about us remain for hours in an approximately unchanging illumination. The changes in colour which they undergo over an extended period, as a result of the shifting position of the sun or of the clouds, take place so gently and so continuously that they are frequently quite imperceptible. During this period we are always looking at objects, so that it is imperative that even when we pay careful attention to them the colours about us remain relatively self-identical, and that they be seen not as accidental properties of objects but as means for the identification of objects. The same holds for our colour experiences in connection with artificial illuminations of varying degrees of absolute intensity. The paper on which we are writing and the

[1] " Hence our previous view of the cerebral cortex . . . must be supplemented. We must recognize that in addition to the optic fibres there are touch fibres terminating in the visual cortex, and that these mediate touch sensations, which in company with visual sensations give rise to visual percepts." H. Munk, *Sitzungsber. d. kgl. Akad. d. Wiss. Berlin*, 50, *phy.-math. Kl.*, 1910, p. 1013 f.

desk at which we are sitting undergo practically no perceptible changes over an extended period of time. It is quite conceivable that even an eye which lacked our adaptive mechanisms would, under such conditions of vision, still be able to apprehend colours as properties of objects, and would in consequence still be able to identify the objects.

Transcending the individual identification of individual objects is the idea that for every object there is a stable colour which can be seen in one particular illumination, when all other factors influencing colour-perception are held constant. How does this idea develop?

Apparently it comes into being as a result of experiences of perceptibly changing illumination, particularly those in which the illumination returns to its starting-point. An object loses in brightness when it is moved away from the window, and regains it when it is moved back. When an object in the hand is moved to and from the light, the to-and-fro movements are accompanied by changes in illumination intensity. In both cases the mutual relatedness of certain illumination intensities and certain colour-impressions usually stands out against the background of an unchanging illumination which comprises the greater part of the visual field. The functional relationship, " specific illumination—specific colour," is not to be understood as implying that one intensity of illumination takes precedence over any other. When we speak of the *genuine* colours of objects we mean more than this functional relationship. The distinction between the stable colour of an object and its genuine colour cannot be made except in terms of normal illumination, the unique characteristics of which have already been discussed in detail.[1]

And now one final question : Are the bonds which tie different illuminations together, or which connect illuminations with the object colours belonging to them, governed by the traditional laws of association, or do they follow other laws ? There are three important

[1] *Cf.* § 16.

respects in which the law underlying this synthesis seems to differ from the traditional principle of association : (1) The elements involved in an associative connection are usually assumed to possess a certain independence and stability. Every element exists in its own right, and because of this very independence is able to enter into any other connection. (2) Elements of quite different nature can be associated with each other. They need manifest no inner reference to each other. The idea of a chair is associated approximately as easily with the idea of a physical principle as with the idea of another chair. The elements of traditional associationism are bound together in a purely external way. (3) If two items are to be associated with each other, they must be presented either simultaneously or successively, in the latter case without too great an interval between them. Now how is it with the associations of the colour-experiences with which we are here concerned ? In the first place, the concept of element has quite a different meaning. One specific illumination is not associated with one specific surface colour. Surface colour and illumination constitute, rather, an indissoluble unity. This connection is not built up through experience, and it cannot be broken, even through abstraction. To every visual field with a particular illumination there belongs a *particular* white, a *particular* grey, etc., and we cannot arbitrarily replace these by the same colours in other degrees of pronouncedness. When one illumination with its corresponding colours becomes associated with another illumination with its corresponding colours, the process is not purely external, for the one illumination with its colours emerges from the other, and merges back into it ; they are both indicators and bearers of each other. They produce the experience of a succession which is in itself meaningful. There is no implication in the traditional principle of successive association that the members of the series are meaningfully bound together. And finally—and here we come to the third point—the succession of colour-impressions is less dependent upon the

factor of time than are the traditional successive associations. Simultaneity cannot be considered as a characteristic of our illumination series. The various members
must not, however, follow upon each other too quickly,
if they are to be apprehended as a series. Even an
association of syllables, for example, ceases under such
conditions to be a series.

In the first edition I introduced the concept of
chain-association in order to emphasize the unique
character of the associative principle operative here.
Such chain-associations confront us in every field of
perception in which constancy phenomena are observable.[1]
Apparent distance and apparent size, apparent position
and apparent form, apparent loudness and apparent
distance of sound source—all give us meaningful serial
combinations according to the principle of chain-
association. As far as the synthesis of illuminations is
concerned, the principle of chain-association is embodied
in the consciousness of one object which undergoes all
the changes in colour. Without such a stable point of
reference the principle of chain-association would probably never have acquired the importance which it now
possesses for human consciousness.

Because of the meaningful character of the series
involved in the synthesis of illuminations, it is possible
for us to interpolate and extrapolate for series which
are given in experience only in fragmentary fashion.
Even illuminations which we have never experienced
before do not appear at first in complete and baffling
isolation, for the meaningfulness of the previously experienced series forms a bridge to connect the new with
the old. In order to avoid misunderstandings, may I
assert explicitly that associations in the traditional sense
of the term may also be formed between one illumination
with the colours belonging to it and another illumination
with its colours. If I see a particular surface colour in
a particular illumination and, close at hand, the same

---

[1] *Cf.* R. Hönigswald, *Die Grundlagen der Denkpsychologie,* 2nd ed.,
Teubner, 1925, p. 136 f.

or another surface colour in another illumination, an external association can be formed between the two impressions. Then if, on a later occasion, I see one of the illuminations with its corresponding surface colour, I can reproduce an image of the other. Such associations have little significance for an understanding of the synthesis of illuminations. They are, however, not entirely without interest for us. It would appear, for instance, that it is easier for us on the basis of a non-normally illuminated visual field to reproduce the colours in a normally illuminated field, than it is for us to effect the opposite type of reproduction.

INDEX OF AUTHORS

INDEX